TIPPING THE BALANCE TOWARDS PRIMARY HEALTH CARE

Tipping the Balance Towards Primary Health Care

Edited by

TOM RATHWELL
Nuffield Institute for Health
University of Leeds

JOANA GODINHO
Public Health Specialist
Bethsada, USA

MARJORIE GOTT
Gott Associates
Groby, UK

Avebury

Aldershot · Brookfield USA · Hong Kong · Singapore · Sydney

© T. Rathwell, J. Godinho and M.Gott 1995

Published by
Avebury
Ashgate Publishing Company
Gower House
Croft Road
Aldershot
Hants GU11 3HR
England

Ashgate Publishing Company
Old Post Road
Brookfield
Vermont 05036
USA

British Library Cataloguing in Publication Data

Tipping the Balance Towards Primary
  Health Care
  I. Rathwell, Thomas
  362.1

ISBN 1 85628 941 9

Library of Congress Cataloging-in-Publication Data

Tipping the balance towards primary health care / edited by
    Tom Rathwell, Joana Godinho, Marjorie Gott.
      p. cm.
    Includes bibliographical references and index.
    ISBN 1-85628-941-9 : $55.95 (approx.)
    1. Rathwell, Thomas, 1944–   . II. Godinho, Joana, 1951–   .
    [DNLM: 1. Primary health Care--organization & administration-
    -Europe. 2. Health Care Reform--Europe. W84.6 T595 1995]
RA427.9T55   1995   94-38123
362.1'094--dc20   CIP

Printed and bound by Athenæum Press Ltd.,
Gateshead, Tyne & Wear.

Contents

Part I
The Agenda for Change

Part II
Country Case Studies

vi

Figures and tables

Contributors

Walter Adrahi
Azores Regional Health
Authority
Azores
PORTUGAL

S Ashton
Dudley Health Authority
Stourbridge
West Midlands
UNITED KINGDOM

Joseba Barroeta
Andalucia School of Public
Health
Granada
SPAIN

Eduardo Briones
Andalucia School of Public
Health
Granada
SPAIN

Chris Buttanshaw
Eastern Health Board
Dublin
IRELAND

Francisco Camino
Andalucian School of Public
Health
Granda
SPAIN

Delfim Cardoso
Abravezes Mental Health Centre
Abravezes
PORTUGAL

Concha Colomer
Valencia Public Health Institute
Valencia
SPAIN

John Daley
Dudley Health Authority
Stourbridge
West Midlands
UNITED KINGDOM

Fred Donohue
Eastern Health Board
Dublin
IRELAND

Rosemary Dun
West Lambeth Health Authority
Lambeth
London
UNITED KINGDOM

Hans Ekman
Bohus County Council
Gotenburg
SWEDEN

Gunilla Fahlstrom
Department of Social Medicine
Orebro
SWEDEN

Fidalgo Freitas
Abravezes Mental Health Centre
Abravezes
PORTUGAL

Rosario Giraldes
School of Public Health
Lisbon
PORTUGAL

Joana Godinho
Public Health Specialist
Bethesda, MD
UNITED STATES

Marjorie Gott
Gott Associates
Groby
Leicestershire
UNITED KINGDOM

Gregor Henderson
West Lambeth Health Authority
Lambeth
London
UNITED KINGDOM

Jose Maria de la Higuera
Andalucia School of Public
Health
Granada
SPAIN

Lennart Holmquist
Department of Social Medicine
Orebro
SWEDEN

Henric Hultin
Health and Medical Services
Alvsborg County Council
Vanersborg
SWEDEN

Anne-Marie Jaarnek
Jamtland County Council
Froson
SWEDEN

Amanda Kemp
North Staffordshire Health
Authority
Stoke-on-Trent
Staffordshire
UNITED KINGDOM

Luka Kovacic
Andrija Stampar School of
Public Health
Zagreb
CROATIA

Lars-Olof Ljunberg
Department of Planning
Blekinge County Council
Karlktrona
SWEDEN

Esteban de Manuel
Andalucia School of Public
Health
Granada
SPAIN

Bertil Marklund
Health and Medical Services
Alvsborg County Council
Vanersborg
SWEDEN

M Marsh
Dudley Health Authority
Stourbridge
West Midlands
UNITED KINGDOM

Carlos Costa Neves
Azores Regional Health
Authority
Azores
PORTUGAL

Alison Norman
North Staffordshire Health
Authority
Stoke-on-Trent
Staffordshire
UNITED KINGDOM

Kaj Norrby
Jamtland County Council
Froson
SWEDEN

Ingrid Pincus
Department of Social Medicine
Orebro
SWEDEN

Luis Puig
Valencia Public Health Institute
Valencia
SPAIN

Tom Rathwell
Nuffield Institute for Health
University of Leeds
Leeds
UNITED KINGDOM

Jesus Rodriguez
Audalucia School of Public
Health
Granada
SPAIN

xii

Jose Salazar
Valencia Public Health Institute
Valencia
SPAIN

Mike Smith
Dudley Health Authority
Stourbridge
West Midlands
UNITED KINGDOM

Olga Solas
Andalucia School of Public
Health
Granada
SPAIN

Pertti Soveri
Borga Health Service
Porvoo
FINLAND

Bo Stencrantz
Jamtland County Council
Froson
SWEDEN

Asta Stenvall
Borga Health Service
Porvoo
FINLAND

Ivan Stipanov
Andrija Stampar School of
Public Health
Zagreb
CROATIA

Anna Swift-Johanisson
Department of Social Medicine
Orebro
SWEDEN

Maryrose Tarpey
West Lamberth Health
Authority
Lamberth
London
UNITED KINGDOM

J Tromans
Dudley Health Authority
Stourbridge
West Midlands
UNITED KINGDOM

Glenn Warren
North Staffordshire Health
Authority
Stoke-on-Trent
Staffordshire
UNITED KINGDOM

James Winoy
Jamtland County Council
Froson
SWEDEN

Jo Wood
Dudley Health Authority
Stourbridge
West Midlands
UNITED KINGDOM

Acknowledgements

There are many to whom we are indebted and without whose contributions this book would not be possible. We are grateful particularly to : Per-Gunner Svensson and Walter Hubrich, Regional Office for Europe of the World Health Organisation who contributed much welcomed technical support; Laura Ayres, late Chair of the health services research committee (COMAC HRS) of the European Union; Paul Baker, the COMAC HRS 'chef-de-file' for the Project; Richard Saltman, Emory University in Atlanta; Keith Barnard and Per-Olof Brogen, Nordic School of Public Health in Gotenburg; and Antonio Carreia de Campos, Joas Sennfelt and Teodoro Briz, School of Public Health in Lisbon.

We wish to thank the Regional office for Europe of the World Health Organisation for financial and technical support; and especially the Commission of the European Communities for granting financial support to the project.

We thank Oxford University Press, publishers of the European Journal of Public Health for permission to reproduce the case studies described in Part II. A special thanks goes to Elaine Garvey and Susanne Hinchliffe without whose valiant efforts this manuscript would not have been possible. Finally we would like to thank all those who played a part in the TTB project; we dedicate to them this product of our collective endeavours.

Tom Rathwell, Joana Godinho, and Marjorie Gott

Part I
THE AGENDA FOR CHANGE

1 Tipping the balance toward primary health care: The agenda for change

Tom Rathwell and Joana Godinho

Introduction

The problems caused by chronic diseases, cancer, ageing, disabilities, and new and rising epidemics such as AIDS and illicit drug consumption are increasingly worrying not only to governments but ordinary individuals. At the same time, there are serious concerns about the efficacy of sophisticated technology and existing health services that rely heavily on hospitals and specialised medicine to confront these problems. It is argued therefore that a better primary health care system is necessary to provide more adequate and efficient solutions to these current health problems.

Technological advances in medical care and increased research into health services issues have contributed to a dramatic rise in expenditure on health care in Europe. For example, in 1987 the countries associated with the Organisation for Economic Cooperation and Development (OECD) on average spent 7.5% of their Gross Domestic Product (GDP) on health (Schieber and Poullier, 1989). This is an increase of 42% over the average expenditure of 5.3% of GDP in 1970. Greater research, technological developments and increased spending on health care has not improved the health of the European people as much as might have been expected. Taking life expectancy at birth as one indication of health of a population, again for OECD countries, one finds that life expectancy at birth has increased from 71.0 in 1970 to 75.8 in 1987 (OECD, 1990). This represents an overall increase of 4.8 years or 6.8 percent. Not a

3

particularly impressive increase given the improvements to health care systems that have taken place during the period.

An explanation for the limited improvement in health status over the years may lie in the fact that a large part of health expenditure in most countries goes on hospital services. It is clear from a perusal of Table 1 that within the European countries listed, there is considerable variation of expenditure on hospital inpatient care. The fact that some spend a smaller proportion of their public health expenditure on inpatient care may be more to do with the pluralistic nature of their health care systems than with any concerted effort to provide an adequately resourced primary health care network. Comparability is also compounded by the fact that there is no internationally agreed definition of what constitutes hospital care, primary health care and public health expenditure. Each country interprets such terms according to their particular situation and/or circumstances.

European countries acknowledge that, however they define and measure these terms, pressures from rising demand for health care which in turn is reflected in increased expenditure, has forced them to examine a range of options for changing the system. This is a common concern for all countries, however differently structured their individual health care systems. A solution to the common problem, pursued by most countries is the development of a better system of primary health care, with a greater emphasis on the twin goals efficiency and effectiveness. A number of strategies are being considered by various countries for achieving these objectives. The common factors linking all the various efforts are the Primary Health Care and Health For All (HFA) methodologies propounded by the World Health Organisation (WHO).

Primary health care and health for all

The World Health Assembly in 1977 endorsed a resolution now known by the slogan 'Health For All by the Year 2000'. This resolution committed the member states of WHO to pursuing, as a social policy goal, steps that would allow their populations to lead socially and economically productive lives. The World Health Assembly Meeting was followed by a joint WHO/UNICEF international conference which resulted in the now famous Declaration of Alma Ata (WHO/UNICEF, 1978). The Declaration committed member states to a particular approach to Health For All based on primary health care (PHC).

4

Table 1
Public expenditure on health by country : 1987
(National currency - millions)

Country	Total	Inpatient Care	Percentage
Austria	83340	15223	18.3
Belgium	297000	68539	23.1
Denmark	35400	*27783	78.4
Finland	22894	11745	51.3
France	336750	185896	55.2
Germany	126930	54498	42.9
Greece	253000	82349	32.5
Iceland	14413	10020	69.5
Ireland	1279	936	73.2
Italy	56110000	29440000	52.5
Luxembourg	15284	4414	28.9
Netherlands	26995	17454	64.6
Norway	40549	*25950	64.0
Portugal	202000	*76000	37.6
Spain	1533600	740000	48.3
Sweden	83752	63212	75.5
Switzerland	*12703	*7143	56.2
United Kingdom	21433	12149	56.7

* = 1986 data

Source: OECD, Health Data File, 1989

The concept of PHC, outlined in the Alma Ata Declaration, stresses the importance of a local first contact service provided by primary physicians in conjunction with other community based health workers.

In this model of PHC, locally based care becomes the foundation and first point of a referral according to an individual's particular needs to a network of increasing complexity and sophistication. PHC is not just medical care; it also embraces a range of health related activities such as good water, proper sanitation, nutrition, the physical environment, together with public information and education on health problems.

A basic prerequisite of the Alma Ata approach to PHC is that it should involve the national and local dimensions of a country's health sector in a range of initiatives designed to strengthen and/or re-orient health care services. The comprehensive nature of the HFA approach to PHC will involve the health sector in seeking, obtaining and sustaining the willing cooperation of agencies in other sectors whose actions could have a beneficial effect on the population's health. Moreover, equal importance is given to community participation in health, not only in the mechanisms for planning and managing services, but also to underline the personal contribution individuals can make to health. The fact that organisation of PHC varies widely between developed countries has been noted by WHO (1986);

> In some countries well coordinated teams form the established and recognised first point of contact with the official health system. In others, access to health care may be through General Practitioners, specialists or nurses, all working alone. In many countries, people belonging to particular social groups or living in particular geographical areas are still without good access to primary health care services, while in other instances preventive and rehabilitative services are less generally available than curative services (p.47).

In addition to differences in levels of, and access to, PHC services between countries, there are also differences of interpretation. Vuori (1984) has remarked on the distinction between primary health care and primary medical care; a distinction which he believes few recognise, (particularly health care workers!). He goes on to argue that no one European country can be complacent about its system; all fall short of the Alma Ata Declaration. Green (1987) endorses these views, and, commenting on the situation in the UK, alleges that the spirit of PHC has been subverted, particularly with regard to health promotion policies.

Member states of the European Region of WHO have taken the global approach to HFA articulated by the Alma Ata Declaration and reformulated it in the form of a European Regional Strategy which was formally adopted in 1980. The Strategy,

> calls for a fundamental change in countries' health policies and urges that very high priority be given to health promotion and disease prevention; that all sectors with an impact on health take positive steps to maintain and improve health; that greater stress be placed on the role individuals, families and communities can play in health development; and that primary care should be the major approach used to bring about these changes (WHO, 1986:1).

The commitment to the broad regional strategy, or common health policy for Europe, was strengthened by the adoption by members states of 38 regional targets, against which they agreed to monitor their progress towards its achievement (WHO, 1985). The targets therefore can be taken as a policy challenge to member states to re-orient their health care systems so that they can satisfy the aforementioned objectives. Indeed these goals are reflected in the 38 targets through six identifiable themes: equity; health promotion; community participation; multi-sectoral cooperation; primary health care; and, inter-nation cooperation.

Research for health for all

International organisations, particularly the European Union and the World Health Organisation, are encouraging countries and research teams to cooperate in studying major knowledge gaps in health. Research priorities such as early detection and diagnosis of cancer, assessment of preventive strategies on AIDS, determining risk factors for older person's loss of autonomy, defining strategies for medical and social care of the disabled or evaluating intervention programmes on illegal drug consumption in school children, must rely heavily on the front-line practitioners and health professionals. It is essential therefore that much of the work on these major issues is undertaken at the PHC level.

Moreover, much more insight is needed into the most appropriate ways of planning, organising, managing, and financing PHC services. International studies which cover a variety of different situations, make use of available scientific knowledge, resources and experience, use different but rigorous comparable methodologies and exchange information, are necessary to increase our knowledge in these aspects.

As part of its effort to support member states work towards the common health policy, the European Regional Office in 1985 began development of a research strategy. The strategy outlined in the document Priority Research For Health For All (WHO, 1988a) emphasises the value of undertaking research projects which generate knowledge about the processes of policy formulation and programme planning and their implementation. A companion document Research Policies for Health For All (WHO, 1988b) sets out the framework for research projects in support of HFA. It was envisaged the research would seek to shed light on three areas:

* health policy and organisational behaviour, especially the relationship between social goals, health policy, need and demand for health, and individual health

* inequities because they continue to persist in spite of a variety of efforts

* community participation and intersectoral collaboration are rarely studied and therefore poorly understood.

Research which would add to the required knowledge base needed for effective HFA would likely have four important characteristics. It would be:

* interdisciplinary in its composition
* comparative in its perspective
* clear in its focus
* exemplary in identifying practical workable solutions.

Origins of tipping the balance

The project 'Tipping the Balance Towards Primary Health Care' (TTB) follows previous efforts to identify common organisational and managerial problems in several European countries. It began as an independent initiative with WHO encouragement and support. It was conceived as an action-oriented research project to improve the organisation, management and quality of local community based health services. The focus of the TTB project from the outset embraced three facets: problem identification and analysis; developing responses and

8

evaluating the results; and sharing the lessons of experience to a wider audience. The overall purpose of TTB was to develop tools and indicators which both promote and monitor change towards the common European policy of health for all based on primary health care in existing systems of health services.

Tipping the Balance was adopted as a slogan, which it was felt embodied several key ideas, and not only the relationship between PHC and hospital care. It was recognised as a slogan which needed to be translated into real local experience. After a series of preliminary discussions, seven European countries (Finland, Ireland, Portugal, Spain, Sweden, United Kingdom and Yugoslavia) agreed to cooperate and collaborate in the project. Fifteen Districts from the seven countries were invited and agreed to participate on the basis of the current status of their PHC development and upon their enthusiasm for mutual cross-national analysis of programme activities and behaviour. Participation carried with it the commitment to assist and encourage each other when implementing their local PHC strategy.

The participating teams started by discussing the essential features of their national health care systems and identifying problem areas in primary health care, which could be the matter for coordinated research at the European level.

Notwithstanding their different health care systems, there were some important problems that repeatedly appeared in most of the districts analyses. These problems revolved around the domination of the hospital as the focus of the medical care system, and the perception of health as a medical problem rather than as a concern and a challenge for a participating community and for all the sectors of the society and economy.

Specifically, participants identified a list of common problem areas, including management issues (appropriate organisation and management of PHC, collaboration between health and health related sectors, financing and budgeting of PHC); development of human resources (managerial skills, intra-professional team work cooperation, and responsiveness to patients); and community participation (education for health, and participation in policy-making, planning and management).

Following the selection of topics of most interest to all districts, participants allocated themselves to each area of study, and conducted discussions around the development of the sub-projects and studies related to these topics.

Participants pointed to three different change strategies necessary to 'tipping the balance' towards PHC:

*   restructuring strategies - managing decentralisation and creating indicators for resource allocating and monitoring in PHC;

*   re-educating strategies - improving interactive skills of PHC workers;

*   and facilitating strategies - increasing community participation.

Although there was variety in the specific focus and entry points adopted by different participating districts, there was a unifying set of linked basic working assumptions underpinning the whole TTB initiative. First, decentralising organisation, management and decision-making competence as near as possible to where services are provided to people will improve the efficiency, quality and sensitivity of services. Secondly, decentralisation requires planning, budgeting and monitoring systems which services its purposes. Thirdly, it calls for mechanisms which enable managers and others to work with the community. This means creating appropriate local forums for debate and decision on health issues; enhancing the interactive skills of health workers; and enabling specific interventions which address major problems and promote the health of the population. The whole TTB project tests the validity of these assumptions.

In 1988 a political decision was taken by the participating districts to seek support for the project from the European Commission (EC) through COMAC HSR Committee. The rigorous procedure necessary to secure EC support has served to sharpen the objectives and the analysis of the project.

The main objective of the TTB project was to clarify and evaluate some potentially relevant and effective organisational models and mechanisms. These , it was hoped, would contribute to Tipping the Balance towards improved provision of primary health care, by conducting experimental studies in three interlinked areas:

a)   decentralisation of primary health care;
b)   indicators for resource allocation and monitoring in PHC;
c)   community participation and interactive skills for PHC workers.

The project also pursued other specific objectives:

*   to describe current levels of organisation and management of local/district-based primary health care services and provide a set

of commonly accepted definitions about primary health care

* to promote the development of locally-based research, by studying local relevant issues with adequate scientific support

* and to create a European network of district-based researchers, who will act beyond the time frame of the project.

PHC planning and organisation is affected by a number of local factors that differ from one setting to another. The methodologies used to solve research questions related to management must take into account these peculiarities. The results of the studies cannot be analysed as if they were a common protocol multi-centred study, but they can be compared and contrasted in order to have a better understanding of the issues, and suggest new hypothesis to be tested by subsequent research.

An innovative approach was used to involve health and health-related professionals who work at the primary health care level, where problems originate and have to be solved daily. Locally-based research teams were assisted by academic institutions with experience in organisational and managerial health services research.

The studies were conducted in a wide range of contexts, utilising a variety of locally determined approaches whilst pursuing the common HFA strategy and goals to achieve improved PHC.

Re-structuring strategies have been the particular focus of two sub-projects within the overall project. These are the inter-linked areas of decentralisation and indicators for resource allocation and monitoring referred to earlier. The two remaining change strategies, re-education and facilitation are the research subject of the third sub-project, community participation and interaction skills. Each of these three sub-projects is now briefly described. A more detailed discussion of each sub-project is given below in Chapters 2-4 respectively.

Sub-project 1 - Managing decentralisation of primary health care

Managing decentralisation of health care was one of the crucial issues identified for investigation by the participants. As PHC focuses on first contact services, provision of effective care at the local level is a priority in all districts. The assumption made is that decentralisation is an effective means to stimulate improvements in the delivery of services, to secure better allocation of resources according to needs, to involve the community and to facilitate the reduction of inequities in health.

The sub-project had three objectives:

* to establish, with a variety of approaches in a wide range of settings, whether the decentralisation process is generally an efficient and effective way of delivering health care and meeting community health needs;

* to identify a range of common features in decentralised systems and contrast and understand their relative significance;

* to assess whether the variety of approaches adopted generate compatible findings which contribute to the achievement of the projects overall aims.

Decentralisation of primary health care was seen by most of the participants as being a necessary prerequisite for its transformation leading to major changes in the roles, responsibilities and relationships of those concerned (WHO, 1988c). A research imperative was that the benefits of decentralisation should be seen to outweigh its disadvantages, otherwise the whole exercise would be judged futile.

Research issues of particular interest to the district teams were:

* the range and types of health care premises used for primary health care, the activities undertaken in these premises, and to whom and how the services were delivered.

* the current costs of providing the service and the manner in which the quality of service was measured.

* the changing pattern of services given to and demanded by different types of patients/clients.

* whether or not primary health care teams existed and the extent to which they were integrated into the primary health care network.

* the scope for improving collaborative relationships with other agencies both within and outside the health sector. An additional factor here is the potential for decentralisation of specialist hospital services and/or resources.

Shedding some light on these questions was considered important for and central to the strategic objectives of moving from a centralised to a decentralised system of PHC. Indeed, studies elsewhere reinforce the importance of these and other questions (Mills, *et al* 1990).

A number of approaches had been adopted. Some participants considered a wide range of system components, to establish the effectiveness or otherwise, of a decentralisation strategy. Others took a more selective approach to highlight those key parts of the decentralisation process which were considered relevant in achieving the overall aims.

Districts also used a variety of methods to test their assumptions; collecting and analysing quantitative data where possible and useful to do so. In other cases, a qualitative approach was utilised as a more appropriate mechanism for illustrating and exploring the decentralisation process.

It is accepted that for decentralisation to be effective close monitoring of changes in the following areas was necessary: referral patterns; morbidity and health inequities; accessibility and utilisation rates; and perhaps most importantly, patient and professional satisfaction. Thus a related area of investigation was the benefits to the user, in terms of accessibility and continuity of care, of a decentralised system of PHC. The districts participating in this sub-project were: Andalusia (Spain); Eastern Health Board (Ireland); North Staffordshire (United Kingdom); Orebro (Sweden); Porvoo (Finland) and Zadar (Yugoslavia).

Sub-project 2 - Indicators for resource allocation and monitoring in primary health care

The development and use of indicators as tools for resource allocation and monitoring at both operational and planning levels was the common central focus of participating districts in this sub-project. Understanding financing and allocating mechanisms, and monitoring the results of these, are important pre-requisites for ensuring that PHC policies become a reality (WHO, 1988c). With this in mind the sub-project had three objectives:

*   to develop and agree appropriate quantity and quality indicators which can be applied to effectively monitor PHC activities, and be useful planning tools for resource allocation responsive to local needs;

*   to provide an opportunity for interchange of ideas and experience

13

on the development and application of indicators relevant to decentralised PHC;

*   to establish whether the use of indicators within a decentralised PHC facilitates resource allocation sensitive to local needs.

Individual district studies assess the process of development and implementation of indicators in a decentralised PHC for resource allocation and monitoring purposes, with reference to five main questions:

*   Can indicators be developed that are of relevance to local decision making?

*   Will monitoring be improved through better integration of resource utilisation, service performance and goal achievement?

*   Which PHC indicators will provide better and appropriate information on PHC performance at both the local and strategic level?

*   What are the relevant factors that influence decentralised planning of PHC?

*   Does decentralisation and the use of appropriate indicators facilitate the development of more locally responsive services?

Planning and budgeting are key components of the management and organisational structure of any health care system, whether or not it is centralised or decentralised. An important feature of planning and budgeting is the processes used to determine the resources to be allocated to health care, the manner in which those resources are to be deployed and for what expected benefit. Thus it could be argued that resource allocation methods are synonymous with planning and budgeting. If this is the case, then resource allocation can be analysed on several levels:

*   within the national and local economy and the way in which allocation decisions at these levels affect the distribution of resources between health and other sectors.

*   within the health sector alone between primary health care and

hospitals and between different aspects or areas of primary health care.

*   within the different areas or strands of primary health care, especially to different groups and localities.

Taking these initial and preliminary thoughts into account, the participating districts identified four specific questions or issues to guide their research: how to design indicators aimed at measuring both quantity and quality? ; how to develop appropriate and acceptable indicators? ; who influences in choice of indicators and to what effect? ; and, what are the main advantages and disadvantages associated with the use of an agreed set of indicators?

It was noted earlier that a key feature of the TTB research was its flexibility allowing each district to employ the research methods and procedures which they considered to be most appropriate. A problem of this approach is, of course, that the different methods used make comparison of the results somewhat difficult. In order to facilitate comparison of the results of the resource allocation sub-project, each participating district was asked to focus on a common investigative framework: financing mechanisms; allocation methods and patterns; and monitoring and evaluating resource use. Four districts took part in this sub-project: Azores (Portugal); Bohus (Sweden); Dudley (United Kingdom); and Jamtland (Sweden).

Sub-project 3 - Community participation and interaction skills

Matching health and welfare provision with the needs of the community is problematic. It is however essential in a changing society to insure the sensitivity of services to local needs especially when resources are static or in relative decline. In order to develop and maximise the impact of these services in primary health care, a well functioning form of participation with the community is a prerequisite.

This sub-project is divided into more specific areas which are united by a common core. The common objectives are threefold:

*   Explore and enhance different ways and methods of involving the communities in the provision of PHC;

*   Analyse and develop different methods of improving PHC sensitivity to communities' needs;

* Establish methods of promoting healthier lifestyles in the community using interactive skills.

Community participation and interaction skills are also equally important requirements for a successful and effective primary health care system (WHO, 1988c). The trouble is that there is very little opportunity for community involvement in health care, at least at the level envisaged by HFA (WHO, 1985), because of a lack of enthusiasm on the part of governments and health care providers (WHO, 1988c).

Public participation has long been a debated issue in the literature on public policy making (Simmie, 1974; Fagence, 1977; Boaden, *et al* 1982; Rathwell, 1987). Most of the debate about participation is cloaked in terms of democratic theory with its attendant issues of representation, power and control. Perhaps the concept of participation most central to the TTB research is the notion of 'partnership' on Arnstein's (1969) ladder of citizen participation. Partnership in this context refers to a situation whereby policies and programmes are determined through a process of negotiation by all parties concerned.

For the purposes of the participating districts, participation was defined as the process of assisting satisfactory bodies to develop and improve services in partnership with the local community. Two alternative models were identified for investigation of whether the democratic involvement of actors from the local community enhances their ability to influence the acceptability and legitimacy of health care services. The alternatives were first those that relied upon informal mechanisms for involving local groups and organisations in the decision making process; and second, those in which participation was formally established through the political process.

It was recognised that particular attention had to be paid to the level of participation in local democracy by different groups in society and their corresponding expectations arising from such involvement. Issues for investigation were the services changes that resulted and their acceptability; policies and programmes that did not progress further and why; and the reaction to increased local democracy among professional providers. An overarching question was whether the participatory mechanisms designed to increase local visibility and legitimacy of PHC led to improvements in equity and effectiveness. Other main areas of focus for the group of districts in this sub-project were:

* Prevention and promotion studies which concentrated on developing and extending the health promotional skills of health

professionals, and building teamwork for successful health promotion. Teamwork in this case meant encouraging and fostering inter-professional working and professional/lay worker collaboration.

* Intersectoral collaboration using a multi-agency approach, thus recognising that a single agency was inappropriate for delivering effective primary health care. The value of developing and using common health protection management protocols was considered very important.

* Re-orientation to PHC was a specific objective of the studies in this section, although it is a common thread running through all the sub-projects. The particular emphasis here was on developing innovative partnerships between hospital, PHC staff and local communities.

Eight districts participated in this sub-group: Alvsborg (Sweden); Blekinge (Sweden); Dudley (United Kingdom); Valencia (Spain); and, Viseu (Portugal).

Conclusion

The project arose from a consensus about a range of problems facing the development of PHC in many European countries. These problems encompass such wide-ranging issues as the continuing dominant perspectives of health, or rather ill-health, as a medical matter and not something which should be the concern of the community and/or society as a whole. There is a challenge here for the health care system to delivery services which are both needed and acceptable to the community. This suggests some form of decentralised health services delivery system and the active and meaningful participation of the local community in determining the nature and pattern of the services to be provided.
Other issues of particular concern identified by the participating districts were the frequent lack of both horizontal coordination and effective collaboration between health workers and delivery institutions in the health care sector, and other sectors allied to health. Communication and cooperation between the PHC system as the first point of contact, and institutions providing specialist care was judged to be poor in most cases. It was acknowledged that what was required was a synergistic

relationship between PHC and specialist care whereby the former is supported by rather than controlled or dominated by the latter.

The three sub-projects are listed separately for operational purposes but the boundaries between them are not clear cut and there are many cross-overs. The case studies described in Part II in this volume clearly illustrate the nature and relationship of the shared common concerns of the project.

The focus of the project was on problem identification and analysis, on developing responses and critically evaluating the results and on sharing the lessons in a manner which will facilitate their adoption by others where appropriate and relevant. The research teams used a variety of methods to assess their suppositions. Some used quantitative methods to collect and analyse data, whereas others employed qualitative mechanisms. Each district applied the investigative procedure it considered most suitable to its requirements.

Taken together the sub-project studies provide a comprehensive overview of different forms of decentralisation and its affect, and of the new roles and responsibilities demanded of professionals and the health care systems. And enables an appreciation by others of the positive and negative impacts on health and health services.

The foregoing discussion set out in broad terms the research agenda of the three sub-projects aimed at 'Tipping The Balance Towards Primary Health Care'. The relative success of the sub-projects can be discerned from the following substantive papers which examine in more detail the three main research themes and indicate the extent to which the participating districts achieved their particular goals. Moreover, further information on each district and their particular approach is provided in the individual case study reports.

2 Managing decentralisation in primary health care

Tom Rathwell

Introduction

Traditionally and historically PHC often has been a poor cousin to the curative-oriented hospital-based services. The Declaration of Alma Ata endeavoured to break the mould of the curative model of health care by encouraging countries to re-orient their health care systems towards a particular concept of PHC. Two hallmarks of this concept are decentralisation and community participation.

Decentralisation is encouraged because the central administration level often is not close enough to the people to understand their particular problems and needs. The model of decentralisation preferred is one whereby

> communities are each given a certain financial ceiling together with the *responsibility* and *authority* use that money ... to develop primary health care in accordance with the programme they have worked out [emphasis added] (WHO, 1978:68-9).

Decentralisation will not be effective without community support and involvement, thus community participation is central to any attempt to decentralise the means of funding and delivering PHC. Community participation is defined by the WHO as the process by which individuals and families assume responsibility for their own health and welfare and for those of the community, and develop the capacity to contribute to their and the community's development (WHO, 1978:50).

It can be argued on the basis of the above that one cannot have effective PHC without first establishing some form of decentralised means for delivering the service and obtaining the commitment and participation of the community. Taking the Alma Ata Declaration at face value, the route to PHC lies down the decentralisation and community participation road.

This chapter describes the approach towards decentralising PHC taken by several countries in Europe, under the rubric of 'Tipping the Balance Towards Primary Health Care'. The important role of community participation in the decentralisation process is not being ignored as it is the subject of separate discussion in Chapter 4. Before embarking on a discussion of the six case studies, it is first necessary to explore in some detail the concept of decentralisation. The discussion then moves to a brief description and analysis of each of the case studies involved in the decentralisation project and the results of the analysis is compared and contrasted with the broad aims of the project. The chapter concludes with an assessment of the lessons drawn from the exercise.

Decentralisation

Decentralisation seems to be one of those over-worked but little understood words which currently are fashionable. It has become a portmanteau term - it takes on different meanings to suit different circumstances. Starting with the dictionary, decentralisation is described as 'to withdraw from the centre: to transform by transferring functions from a central government, organisation or head to local centres', which tells us something but not very much.

Cheema and Rondinelli (1983) identify four models of decentralisation: deconcentration; delegation; devolution; and transferral.

*   Deconcentration - the redistribution of administrative responsibilities only within the existing structure of central government. What this amounts to is a shifting of workload from centrally located offices to agencies in the field but these agencies have no authority to make decisions or to exercise discretion. Thus power is still held centrally.

20

*   Delegation - the transferral to or the creation of a broad authority to plan and implement decisions relating to particular activities, without direct supervision by a higher authority. Note, however, that this form of delegation relates only to specified tasks and not to all activities. Central government retains overall responsibility for the actions of its 'delegates'.

*   Devolution - governments or agencies relinquish certain functions to new or different organisations which are outside their direct control. Devolved organisations usually exhibit four characteristics:

  -     Local units are autonomous and independent;
  -     Clear and defined geographical boundaries;
  -     Corporate status and power to secure resources;
  -     Reciprocal, mutually beneficial relationships with the central body.

*   Transferral - the handing over of responsibility or 'selling' of assets by the central government to a non-governmental institution to operate and manage. The non-governmental body may be a private company or organisation, or a voluntary agency. All 'rights' are transferred to these non-government agencies and central government no longer takes a direct interest in the way in which they function.

Malcolm (1989) re-interprets and re-labels Cheema and Rondinelli's four models of decentralisation as deconcentration, devolution, corporatisation and privatisation. This is not a refinement of the terminology surrounding the process of decentralisation, rather an attempt to find labels which appear to fit the New Zealand context.

Decentralisation therefore can and does take several forms. This issue will be returned to later with consideration of the approaches and results of decentralisation in the six experimental sites. Of particular interest will be which of the four models described above have been adopted or adapted by the six districts. However, before doing so, It is necessary to consider the rationale for decentralisation, and in particular: what makes decentralisation such an attractive alternative to existing methods of managing large public sector organisations?

Peters and Waterman (1982) did not start the decentralisation bandwagon but they certainly can be said to have given the concept an important boost, especially in the public sector with the publication of their book In Search of Excellence. Although they identified several attributes which distinguish a successful company from the less successful, the notion of the importance of getting 'close to the customer', had particular appeal to those in the public sector and especially in the health care arena. In this context, it can be postulated that 'getting close to the customer' is itself a form of decentralisation. Indeed, according to Cheema and Rondinelli (1983) there are important benefits to be derived from decentralisation:

* It enables policies and plans to be tailored to the needs of local people;

* Officials are able to develop a better understanding of local problems and needs which in turn means that they have a better information base on which to formulate realistic and effective plans;

* It gives the local officials an opportunity to develop and enhance managerial skills;

* It can lead to a more flexible, innovative and creative administration which is much less bureaucratic and responds more quickly.

* It is a way of involving local people, especially ethnic and/or minority groups in decision making;

* Local understanding should in turn lead to a more equitable distribution of resources especially to those in greatest need.

* Officials can more effectively locate and monitor services within local communities if they are a part of that community, or at least, close to it.

A different perspective of decentralisation is given by Hoggett and Hambleton (1987) who argue that it is now well-established in the public sector. They put forward three reasons in support of their view: first, that what may have started as a fad is now so widely adopted that it is now considered to be established practice. Second, it is managerially attractive in terms of greater cost efficiency and effective use of resources. And third, recent technological advances, especially in the fields of information and communication technology, have made decentralisation to not only possible but easy to implement. Hoggett and Hambleton eschew the distinctions of decentralisation espoused by Cheema and Rondinelli, instead arguing that in the public sector there are only two observable approaches to decentralisation; consumerist or collectivist.

The consumerist approach 'gives primary emphasis to enhancing the responsiveness of local government service provision' (Hoggett and Hambleton, 1987: 18), embracing such things as listening to the consumer, becoming more accessible to the consumer, and speaking to the consumer. All part of the edict of 'getting close to the customer'. However, for Hoggett and Hambleton the consumerist approach does not go far enough because, although public sector organizations are now very concerned about responding to the wishes of consumers, the approach confers no power or rights to the consumer. They have no say over the decisions, policies, or plans made ostensibly on their behalf.

The collectivist approach 'gives primary emphasis to the democratisation of local government service provision' (Hoggett and Hambleton, 1987:18), and thus has as its avowed objective to empower the consumer, to give them control over the decisions affecting service provision. The consumerist approach is rejected because there is an imbalance in the public service between those who serve and those who are served. The latter have very little or no power of influence over those who make decisions about their services. Also, services are not just provided to an individual but more realistically they are provided to groups of consumers such as, children and the elderly. Thus services are provided and consumed on a collective basis which renders the consumerist or individual approach to service provision, fraught with danger.

What then is the purpose of decentralisation? Arnold and Cole state that the 'overriding objective of decentralisation (is) to make services more responsive' (1987: 137). This suggests that the exercise has more to do with 'getting close to the customer' than any real attempt to give the consumer greater power over the range and nature of provision of public services.

The whole approach to decentralisation, at least in Britain, is best exemplified by the two following quotes from Arnold and Cole (1987):

> The switch to patch or neighbourhood base work has

occurred in many authorities without any deeper perception of the principles of decentralisation' (p 145);

Decentralised provision has not signalled the demise of central and hierarchical management (p 146).

The picture presented by Arnold and Cole (1987) is one in which decentralisation is no more than tokenism because real power to take decisions unencumbered has not accompanied the decentralisation edict. This is not a view shared by the WHO. It sees decentralisation as an important mechanism for generating greater coordination of services and for responding to the needs of local people through the delegation of responsibility, authority and resources to the community (WHO, 1980). Mills and colleagues (1987) wholeheartedly support the position of WHO, by advocating decentralisation as a way of encouraging and obtaining community participation in health care and also promoting local responsibility for health.

The implication of all this is that decentralisation equals a more efficient and effective approach to the provision of health care; whether at the primary, secondary and/or tertiary level (Godinho, 1990). In Britain, it has been argued that the decentralised model provides the opportunity for the principles of delegation, responsiveness and accountability - the so-called hallmarks of general management - to be taken down to the lowest possible level (Daley, 1987). Decentralisation is also on the political agenda for the New Zealand health services, including the possible restructuring of the way in which PHC is managed and funded through devolution to district or community committees (Malcolm, 1989). Scarpaci traces the rationale in logic behind the moves toward primary care decentralisation in certain Latin American countries. He argues that the movement towards decentralisation in the health care sector is gathering pace because, 'where promises of efficiency and tax savings are coupled with prospects for a healthier population decentralisation is politically attractive to the State'(1991: 104).

In short, different countries are attracted to decentralisation for different reasons and have quite different expectations regarding the outcome or effect of such measures. This begs the question of whether or not countries with very different political systems and structures for providing primary health care, collectively, can pursue the common goal of decentralisation, in a coordinated and agreed fashion. The next section briefly describes the approaches to decentralisation occurring in the countries involved in the TTB project through a common framework and set of objectives. The assumption that decentralisation is beneficial underpins the case studies and they set out to test the assertion that decentralisation is necessary 'as a way to stimulate action and change, to establish local targets, to allocate resources according to needs, to involve the communities, and generally to reduce iniquities in health'(Godinho, 1990:43).

Tipping the balance - managing decentralisation of PHC

The Tipping the Balance project was divided into three sub-projects, of which one was Managing Decentralisation. The over-riding concerns of this project were coordination, integration and equity. The sub-project sought to establish and examine the elements and mechanisms of decentralisation, identifying what works, in what areas, in what connections and with what consequences and limits. The central study issue was the empowering of local PHC through:

- Decentralising strategic policy;
- Decentralising budgets, examining accountability, effective allocation and means of facilitating re-allocation.

Within these main objectives, there was also concern in the sub-project with a number of secondary issues:

- Organisational mechanisms of decentralisation;
- Service outcomes affecting continuity, quality, and cost-effectiveness of care;
- Impact on particular target groups, especially the elderly and de-institutionalised mental patients; and
- Educating health care professionals on PHC cooperation.

The countries and districts participating in this sub-project were: Andalucia - Spain; Eastern Health Board - Ireland; North Staffordshire - United Kingdom; Orebro - Sweden; Porvoo - Finland; and Zadar - Yugoslavia.

A form of decentralisation was undertaken in these districts as part of a process to improve and strengthen their respective primary health care systems. The process was being evaluated from two perspectives - that of managers and of consumers - with respect to attitudes, utilisation, accessibility, decision-making, and needs.

Sub-project study areas

This section presents a short synopsis of the studies undertaken as part of the sub-project on decentralisation. Some studies were more advanced than others but all made good progress towards their respective research goals. Each study is now discussed in turn. For more details about the districts and their particular approaches, readers are referred to the specific case studies in Part II of this volume.

The *Andalucia* study was an evaluative one which compared two rural (Basic Health) areas of the province of Seville, before and after the implementation of the new decentralised, primary health care programme. The study had two stages. The first step was to determine the evaluative model and the components to be used in the study. The second phase was to analyse the decision-making processes taking place in each area and at different levels in order to identify the factors both conducive to and inhibitive of change. Although it was not the original intention, it transpired that the new reforms were introduced and monitored in one area but not in the other. Thus one of the areas provided a control against which to measure the effectiveness of the reforms. A consequence of this was that the 'reform' area was given priority in the allocation of additional resources, whereas the 'control' area did not benefit from extra resources.

The organisational structure differed between the two areas. In the 'reform' area health professionals were integrated into primary care teams under the direction of the Basic Area Director. In the 'control' area, administrative responsibilities were split between the local and regional authorities, and the professionals tended to work individually. The differentiation with regard to resources meant that in the 'control' area the pattern and nature of the services available remained largely unchanged. In the 'reform' area the extra resources resulted in an increase in facilities and services with a re-orientation towards the needs of the population.

The crucial question was, has a decentralised form of primary health care been more beneficial to the inhabitants of the 'reform' area? This was a difficult question to answer but from surveys conducted in both areas it seems that there was little difference with regard to their perceptions of the 10 most important health services. The 'reform' area had a greater awareness and knowledge of local PHC services and tended to make greater use of the available services. Significantly perhaps, those in the 'reform' area were of the opinion that they received a better quality PHC service than did their counterparts in the 'control' area.

A conclusion which can be drawn from the Andalusian study is that decentralisation of the management structure of PHC down to the local level does appear to produce positive benefits for the recipients of the service; benefits not reflected in more centralised approaches.

The aim of the *Eastern Health Board* project was to provide an effective and efficient delivery of health services to the Board's population. The also study had two parts: the first dealt with the reorganisation of the Health Board into six districts based around general hospitals. The second explored further the concept of decentralised management of health services in localities with an emphasis on community participation, and health promotion. The project was not fully completed within the timescale allotted to the European Commission funded programme. Nevertheless, particular progress can be reported.

The first stage has been completed with the Health Board being split into 45 localities (approximate population 27,000) centred around six districts, each based on a general hospital. These localities form the focus of the Board's activities. It is expected that the primary health care staff will be responsible for measuring need, allocating resources and monitoring activities and outcomes at the locality level, although final approval for the development is still awaited.

The second part of the study focused on one district and sought to develop models of decentralised management with an emphasis on community participation and health promotion. A supplementary aspect of the study was to develop an information system for localities which would facilitate equitable and efficient delivery of services.

The decision to proceed with this reorganisation awaits approval from Central Government. However, progress was made in experimenting with the proposed localities. Localities containing areas with the highest Standardised Mortality Ratios (SMRs) were selected and the local Directors of Community Care were asked to identify the resources available within the localities, to identify a medical officer for the locality and plan an integrated programme for health promotion. The plans have been prepared and different aspects of the locality management system are being piloted in the 'Community Ward' scheme for the elderly.

While the overall aim of the Eastern Health Board proposal is directed towards decentralisation, much of the detail associated with this is discussed more fully in the following chapters on resource allocation and community participation.

The *North Staffordshire* project had three aims: to evaluate the introduction of decentralised management structures on the delivery of PHC services; to consider whether the benefits of decentralisation outweigh its disadvantages; and to assess whether decentralised management structures enhance the quality of PHC services.

The work undertaken was to assess the extent to which a decentralised management structure had produced perceived benefits, at least as far as those involved in the organisation change were concerned. An audit of the organisational climate for decentralisation was undertaken using the HAY questionnaire. This is a technique designed to measure attitudes - what people really feel/believe is occurring within the organisation. In particular the audit was designed to answer two important questions:

*   Has locality Management in North Staffordshire moved decision making from a centralised to a decentralised base?

*   Does decentralisation truly facilitate services that are responsive and appropriate to local communities?

The results of the audit among senior staff of the community health services unit confirmed that there was widespread support for and commitment to decentralisation. The establishment of locality management was seen as having been an imaginative step. One which was innovative, gave individuals responsibility and, overall, was perceived to have shifted decision making to such an extent that the services provided were in response to the needs of the local community. The audit has confirmed that decentralisation can be a powerful tool provided the organisation concerned is truly committed to making itself more responsive to the wishes of the population it seeks to serve. From the point of view of the service providers, the decentralisation of the community services was judged to be successful, although the providers were not as satisfied with the restructuring as were managers. Perceived benefits for the staff of decentralisation were, among others, personal development, teamwork and trust, adult treatment, and service reputation. Thus from a management/provider perspective, the decentralisation of community health services was judged a success.

The aim of the *Orebro* scheme was to create greater possibilities for local inhabitants and PHC personnel to influence the formulation of policy for local health care services and to influence the implementation of such policy. This would lead, it was hoped, to more effective decision making.

As a result of new legislation introduced in 1986, Orebro county decided to experiment with local PHC committees in four districts while in a fifth district responsibility for PHC was devolved to the municipality

- a radical departure from existing practice. The objectives of the two experiments were: to improve collaboration between services which in turn was expected to lead to a better service for the public and improved efficiency, and to extend the possibilities for citizen participation thus strengthening local democracy.

The PHC committees consisted of appointed politicians who were to be responsible for budgets, planning, and monitoring. In each case, someone undertook the responsibility for administrating the committee's work supported by clerical staff. The work of the committees was monitored and evaluated over a period of two and a half years. The results of the evaluation suggest that the original objectives of the experiment - democracy and efficiency - were only partially achieved.

The aim to increase democracy in the decision making process was generally unsuccessful with very few people aware of the existence of the PHC committee. Moreover, people did not view the committee as having any power or influence instead stating that if they wished to raise or influence an issue they would contact the chief medical officer or someone on the PHC staff. The staff themselves did not view the committee as having any impact on the way that they provided services to the local population. The politicians on the other hand felt that they had a useful and meaningful role to play.

The experiment did seem to lead to greater efficiency as the senior staff (chief medical and nursing officers) reported greater freedom to carry out their tasks along with an increased workload. They gained increased responsibilities and authority which in turn enabled them to exercise greater control over local PHC issues.

The existence of local political committees in principle did increase possibilities for local participation if not in fact. The experiment could be considered successful even though the local PHC committees played a supportive role to the senior PHC staff rather than an initiating role.

The aim of the *Porvoo* study was to strengthen PHC by moving it closer to the community, and enhancing ties with the municipal administration combined with an increased delegation of budgetary and administrative responsibilities. A supplementary aim was to test the assumption that decentralising PHC has a positive effect over outputs and outcomes.

The PHC services in Porvoo have been split into eight smaller integrated units or 'cells'. Each unit or 'cell' serves a geographic area with a population of 3500-7000. The units or 'cells' have the responsibility and authority to provide primary medical care services, preventive health care, home nursing services and services for schools.

Each unit had a defined functional and financial framework and was expected to operate within it.

The effects of the organisational changes were evaluated against seven criteria: continuity of care; services coverage; accessibility of services; consumption of services; morbidity; patient satisfaction; and worker satisfaction. The evaluation process showed that continuity of care had increased and improved, and that health care personnel were more satisfied with working in a decentralised environment.

The aim of the *Zadar* study was to assess the efficiency, efficacy and accessibility of existing health care services and the effect upon the quality of care provided. The research had three tasks:

* An appraisal of and improvement in accessibility and utilisation of existing services;

* An assessment of communication systems between different levels and types of PHC; and

* An investigation of the interface between primary and secondary health care.

With respect to the first task, data was gathered on spatial and temporal distance to PHC services, working hours of the PHC teams, choice of service and organisation of emergency health care. The focus of task two was on the relationships and the factors which influence them, between occupational health, general practice, school medicine and dental health care. The third task concentrated on collecting data which would permit the identification and resolution of problems in communication between the two levels.

Progress on this project was patchy, with studies of the utilisation of health care and the flow of patients within the district only recently completed.

Discussion

It is difficult to give an adequate assessment of the outcome of each project given that they were at different stages of completion when the research project ended. It is possible, however, to comment on the projects: first, in terms of what they have tried to do (that is, the type or form of decentralization being pursued); and second, to evaluate the relevant extent of their success.

30

With respect to the first issue - type of *decentralisation* - Table 2 assesses the decentralisation approach adopted by the various areas, according to the taxonomy of Cheema and Rondinelli (1983). As the table demonstrates, some of the studies appear to embrace some of the attributes of two types of decentralisation and therefore the placing according to the criteria of each category is less precise for some than it is with others. In three cases (North Staffordshire, Orebro and Porvoo) it appear that the model of decentralisation being followed was that of devolution whereby considerable power and autonomy was invested in the decentralised structure. The remaining three cases seemed to favour a more hybrid model of decentralisation, starting with deconcentration and moving towards delegation (Easter Health Board and Zadar) or beginning with delegation and moving towards devolution (Andalucia). A common feature of these latter three studies is that, in some aspects, there appears to be a considerable degree of central control over the activities of the decentralised units. This assertion may be ill-founded, in that the reports available on progress so far gives little information about the structural changes either contemplated or implemented. As the implementation period for many of the projects extends beyond the life of the research, only time will tell which model of decentralisation has been adopted, and why.

As there is some ambiguity over the approach taken by the different case studies to decentralisation, perhaps the outcome or collective success of the process will be easier to discern. The stated common objectives of all the case studies are: empowerment; collaboration; equity; re-orientation; re-structuring; responsiveness; skills; and, participation. The success of each project according to these stated objectives is depicted in Table 3. A discussion of each of these attributes now follows.

Empowerment generally means giving to others the means or facilities to enable them to exercise choice or control over those things which affect their normal activities. This can be taken in at least two ways: by giving staff greater information and autonomy over how they discharge their responsibilities; and/or by enabling people - the recipients of the service -to have greater influence and involvement in the packages of services provided. In the context of these studies of decentralisation it is the latter aspect of empowerment which is taken as the crucial test. Unfortunately, it is unclear from the way in which the case studies were undertaken whether they took this view of empowerment or whether they had the former concept in mind. Although empowerment was not an explicit aim of the case studies it may well have been an implicit goal, it is clear from the results that the greater the community's involvement

31

Table 2
Models of decentralisation

Type of decentralisation

	Project	Deconcentration	Delegation	Devolution	Transferral
Andalucia		-	x———————	—x	-
Eastern Health Board		x———————	—x	-	-
North Staffordshire		-	-	x	-
Orebro		-	-	x	-
Porvoo		-	-	x	-
Zadar		x———————	—x	-	-

32

Table 3
Outcome of decentralisation

Case study projects

	Andalucia	Eastern Health Board	North Staffs	Orebro	Porvoo	Zadar
Empowerment	-	-	-	-	-	-
Collaboration	*	*	*	*	*	x
Equity	-	*	-	-	-	-
Re-orientation	*	*	*	*	*	x
Restructuring	*	*	*	*	*	*
Responsiveness	-	*	*	*	*	x
Skills	-	x	x	x	x	x
Participation	*	*	*	-	-	-

- = Not explicit goal

* = Achieved, or working towards

x = Not achieved, results incomplete

in PHC the greater the opportunity for their empowerment.

Collaboration can have many connotations but it is generally taken to mean working together with shared or joint responsibility. Using this working definition, it is apparent from Table 3 that, where the information is given, most projects were successful in improving and strengthening collaborative arrangements and procedures. Decentralisation does seem to lead to a closer working relationship with other agencies, but it is not without its problems (Law, 1990). From the evidence presented in the case study reports it is not clear that the perceived benefits of close cooperation and collaboration will be sustained for the foreseeable future. Although the evaluation exercise undertaken in North Staffordshire does suggest that possibly one can be sanguine on this aspect.

Equity is normally defined as fairness and in health care terms this is taken to mean providing services according to needs. Little information is available from the case studies regarding their respective approaches to this issue. Only one project (Eastern Health Board), had given specific attention to the equity question and even then their progress was incomplete. This seems to be an issue in which there is common cause but very little clear understanding of what to do or how to do it. There may have been an assumption on the part of the districts that equity was an implicit element in all the projects, but there was little evidence to suggest that it was given special attention.

Re-orientation in the context of the projects means shifting the emphasis, in health care terms, from hospitals to primary health care. The success of the studies in achieving this outcome was difficult to assess as little information was available from the case-study reports. However, from the preliminary information given this was a stated long term objective and all the projects do appear to be working towards its achievement.

Re-structuring can have a variety of meanings but in this context it is defined as changing the structure of the health care organisation such that, through decentralisation, decision making is taken down to the lowest level possible within the organisation. This may mean that a different structural arrangement is necessary in order to achieve this objective. It is clear from this therefore that re-structuring can take several different forms. It is evident from Table 3 that re-structuring was a common feature of all the projects, and a major feature of the exercise.

Responsiveness embraces three strategies: listening to the consumer; increasing consumer accessibility; and, speaking to the consumer

(Hoggett and Hambleton, 1987). This essentially 'consumerist' approach is the one followed by the study areas. Only one of the projects (Orebro) clearly stated that one of the aims was to 'strengthen local democracy' through the process of decentralisation. However, despite the best of intentions the project evaluators found that local democracy did not improve as a result. The other projects did not appear to entertain ambitions of enhancing the decision making process through giving the local population a say, rather they set their sights on greater awareness of local needs and to using this awareness when formulating policies and plans for meeting these needs.

Skills is the one aspect of the studies about decentrialisation in which there was little information to be discerned from the reports. Skills as it is understood within the overall context of the studies means improving the interactive expertise of primary health care workers and other staff. Very little information about this was available from the reports, and those that do comment on this objective seem to see it as a side-effect of decentralisation, referring only to the impact of the change on workers. However, it may be that skill change was so bound up with the process of change that it was not thought necessary to treat it as a separate issue.

Participation can take place on two levels at least in a public sector organisation: involving workers in the decision making process, and involvement of the wider community. Both concepts of participation were pursued by the studies but not necessarily together in any one. Participation can take a variety of meanings and it appears from the case study reports that different projects were applying different definitions. None, however, seem to be trying for full participation which Pateman states as 'a process where each individual member ... has equal power to determine the outcome of decisions' (1970:71). The projects which commented on their efforts to encourage greater participation generally were less ambitious than this. They tended to go for 'partial participation' in which those who are party to the decision have some influence over the final outcome, but such influence is only partial because ultimately the final say in the matter rests with one party or person.

Conclusion

Decentralisation is a two way process - it requires political will at the centre to shift from central control through deconcentration to devolution, and it requires commitment and courage at the local level to open up to the community at large the processes by which services are determined

35

and delivered.

The case studies demonstrate that the concept of decentralisation has been interpreted and applied differently in each case. This difference of view about decentralisation can be taken as a demonstration of the robustness of the concept and not necessarily a weakness of understanding. The rationale for decentralisation (common to all the projects) can be stated as:

*   a mechanism for generating and sustaining change
*   improves and strengthens organisational processes
*   leads to better quality and more appropriate services
*   fosters and promotes community awareness and involvement

If these are acceptable as the fruits of decentralisation, then the six case studies can be judged to be a success, even though they were at different stages of the evaluation process when the research project came to an end. The outcomes suggest that the decentralised model which most of the projects favoured was devolution - the transferral of a considerable degree of autonomy and, where appropriate, resources down to the local level. The benefits of this approach do appear to be greater and enhanced moral amongst staff, development of and improvement in skills, and greater continuity and acceptability of care for the users of the services. On these criteria alone decentralisation is a valid and effective management strategy for securing better quality and more appropriate PHC. There are risks associated with decentralisation, nonetheless, the one observation that can be drawn from these case studies is that while the risk may be great, the rewards are even greater.

3 Indicators for resource allocation and monitoring in primary health care

Rosario Giraldes and John Daley

Introduction

The work undertaken within this sub-project focused upon indicators for funding allocation and services monitoring within the context of the overall TTB initiative. Studies in individual countries addressed specific areas; a common aspect of each being the development and use of indicators both to assess the quality and quantity of provision and as a basis for equitable resource allocation and efficient use of financial and other resources.

In seeking to achieve efficient and responsive PHC services, measurement of resource usage and impact on health is imperative to inform the decision making process. The participants contributing to the sub-project have addressed these issues which in the areas concerned have provoked discussion and provided a foundation on which further work of a comparative nature within and between countries could be undertaken. Important lessons about the development and application of indicators were identified which should assist in any future work on the planning and budgeting of PHC.

Resource allocation in a public health system

There are two main alternative principles for resource allocation in a public health system: one based on equity and the other on efficiency. The basic tenet of the equity principle is that resources should be allocated in such a way that no one is unduly disadvantaged by the distribution. The efficiency principle holds that resources should be distributed in such a way as to ensure the greatest value for the available money. The relationship between the equity and the efficiency principles is outlined in Table 4.

However, if the efficiency principle has a common universal interpretation of outcome maximisation for fixed resources, the equity principle leads to multiple conceptual interpretations depending upon the values of people who use the resources (Le Grand, 1988).

Increasingly more health systems are adopting either explicitly or implicitly, an equity principle as an objective through public intervention in health services provision. Such an approach is being adopted in countries with such different health care systems as those of the United Kingdom, Sweden, Canada and the United States of America [in relation to Medicare and Medicaid] (McGuire, Henderson and Mooney, 1988).

Since the early 1980s health economists in the United Kingdom have taken a central role in seeking to define and clarify the equity principle. Le Grand and Mooney are two who have made a valuable contribution to this process. Le Grand (1982) identified five main types of equity that may be considered as desirable objectives for the allocation of public expenditure: equality of final outcome; equality of use (equal treatment for equal need); equality of private cost; equality of access; and equality of outcome.

Mooney (1983), in considering the allocation of public expenditure, identified seven possible aspects: equality of expenditure per capita; equality of inputs (resources) per capita; equality of input for equal need; equality of (opportunity of) access for equal need; equality of utilisation for equal need; equality of marginal met need; and equality of health.

Le Grand (1988), more recently argues that a distribution is equitable if it is the outcome of individuals making choices under equal constraints. That is, the disparities in health status which result from fully informed individuals exercising preferences with the same range of choices over health and health related activities are not inequitable; but the disparities in health that can be directly related to differences in the constraints facing those individuals are inequitable.

This concept, which is very interesting, is difficult to put in practice in the allocation of health resources as Le Grand himself admits. Other health economists for example, McGuire, Henderson and Mooney (1988), and Culyer (1980), have drawn attention to Rawls (1972) theory of justice as offering a possible solution to the problem by considering the role of justice in individual utility functions, and especially those relating to health care provision.

Table 4
Comparative analysis of alternatives of resource
allocation in a public health system

	Allocation based on an equity principle	*Allocation based on a technical efficiency principle*
Concept	The equity principle usually corresponds to equality of inputs per capital for equal need.	The technical efficiency principle aims to an increase of productivity (for instance it increases the use of beds and better utilisation of available human and material resources.
Scope	It is based on the population needs in a a certain region or district.	It is not based on the population to be served and centred on the provider of health services.
Methods of needs evaluation	The needs evaluation is based, for example, on the age structure of the population; the sex structure of the population; the fertility rate; the health situation (SMR); the level of coverage by health services.	It is not related to need evaluation.
Methods of needs reallocation	The structure of expenditure determined according to the process of need evaluation is applied to the available total expenditure. The difference between the ideal distribution of expenditure and the real one gives origin to increase or decrease rates fixed according to the desired goals.	It compares levels of productivity within services with the same characteristics

39

This work focuses on the 'maxmin' theory; that is , pursuing the idea that a 'just' solution is to maximize the benefit to the least advantaged. This is based on the assumption that such individuals would want to improve their own lot most especially if they happened to be the worst off in society. The benefits sought being defined as primary social 'goods' (for example, income and wealth, basic liberties, and the social basis of self-respect). Even if health care is not expressly mentioned, it can argued that it is included within these aspects.

Pereira (1988), applied the Sen basic capabilities theory to the health sector and suggests that one's health state or status depends on the 'functioning capability' that the individual possesses: (such as, capacity to work, to enjoy free time, etc.). These capacities being directly determined by access to, for example, health services, education and adequate nutrition. In addition there are 'environmental factors' and 'personal characteristics'. Equality of capacities implies equal access to health and supports the concept of equity of access.

Such a conceptual view as this leads towards the utopian, when all the 'goods' which affected health would be equally distributed, with no differentiation according to class, level of income, or education. There are well known differences in the level of health between different socioeconomic groups and the different capacities of the groups to take initiatives to contact health services (Maynard, 1981). Additionally, due to the specific characteristics of health services provision with resource use determined by clinicians and professionals and the range of available services not well known by the consumer makes this an inadequate theoretical framework for an intervention in resource allocation in the health care sector.

If one accepts the premise inherent in the foregoing, then there may be a strong case for positive discrimination. This implies adopting a concept of equity of access for equal need, which, with regard to the primary health care services, should lead towards equity in use of health services. This would mean the active intervention of health care services in the community to meet the need of high risk groups and make possible an equilibrium between supply and demand, which is implicit in this concept of equity.

The equity principle in the allocation of health expenditure

Most governments have devised a mechanism for allocating public sector resources to health care. For illustrative purposes, the methods used in the United Kingdom and Portugal for allocating health care resources are discussed. Since space does not permit a detailed examination of the allocation mechanisms employed by all the countries involved in the TTB project. The United Kingdom and Portugal were chosen because they focus on different components of the health care system.

The United Kingdom: The methodology used for the allocation of financial resources to the health system was that devised in 1976 by the Resource Allocation Working Party (RAWP) (DHSS, 1976). The Working Party's proposals apply to England only, with similar procedured being followed in Scotland, Wales and Northern Ireland. The discussion which follows deals primarily with England, though the relevant points do apply elsewhere in the United Kingdom.

Maynard and Ludbrook (1983) reviewed the different proposals and concluded that in all of them the same broad principle was adopted: namely, basing the resource allocation process on the population size, weighted with standardized mortality ratios (SMRs) to reflect the relative need for services in different parts of each country. At the same time, the authors concluded that differences existed; for example, in the methods of weighting the population, the health services that were to be included in the formula allocations, and in the application of SMRs.

The RAWP formula in use since 1976 has received only slight changes in England, though it has continued to be the focus of much attention, by both politicians and by academics. Indeed, several criticisms have been made of this method of resource allocation.

First of all, PHC services were not included in the RAWP formula, its focus being hospital and community services. According to Maynard and Ludbrook (1983), the exclusion of PHC services reflected the independent contractual status of doctors and other professionals in this sector, and the perceived need to finance such services separately. Furthermore, the general inapplicability of death rates (SMR) to primary care was also a consideration.

A second criticism concerned the absence of specific recognition in the RAWP formula of the part that social factors play in the need for health care. Recently the NHS Management Board has made proposals to include in the RAWP resource allocation formula a measure of social deprivation using British census data (DHSS, 1988).

A third area of disquiet related to the centres of excellence in the NHS; the major teaching and research institutes. Maynard and Ludbrook (1983) argued that the higher costs of teaching hospitals should be taken into account due to the need to maintain national and international centres of excellence. Whilst the RAWP formula acknowledged the differential costs of operating teaching and non-teaching hospitals, the criticism centred on whether the formula adequately reflected the additional costs

41

involved.

Finally, another criticism concerned the process of reallocation of capital expenditure between regions in the English NHS. Buxton and Klein (1978) were early commentators on the specific problems faced by RAWP when related to capital expenditure; through mainly, the formula not taking into full consideration the unequal distribution of capital stock (buildings and equipment) and the absence of any definitive measures of the quality of that capital stock.

Portugal: If the methodology applied in the United Kingdom has been criticized for not including PHC services, the opposite criticism can be made in the Portuguese case, for not considering hospital services.

Giraldes (1987) has tested the use of the financial criteria proposed for PHC services, based on the principles of equity, to the hospital services. Currently, financing of hospital services is based on principles of efficiency and not equity. In fact, Giraldes concluded that the efficiency principle existing in the financing of the hospital services could be combined with a maximum financial target defined, for each district, according to an equity principle.

The second criticism made of RAWP methodology - that of not taking into consideration the social factors underpinning the need for health care has been addressed in the Portuguese approach. An income indicator has been included as a complement to the health situation criteria, thereby allocating more money to districts with lower average income levels.

The third criticism of the RAWP methodology - the cost consequences of funding centres of excellence - does not apply, in the Portuguese case, to the financing of PHC services. The level of care, in this type of service, may be generally considered as uniform throughout the country, and as a consequence it does not make sense to designate (say) urban centres of excellence. If any correction has to be made it would be possibly in an inverse sense, since the offer of consultations in urban hospital settings covers an important part of the demand for PHC services.

Reallocation of capital expenditure has not been considered in the Portuguese case, mainly because of institutional reasons. As in a number of country settings, the allocation of capital and revenue resources is handled separately, and co-ordination of policies not yet fully developed.

There are three main resource allocation criteria used in PHC in Portugal, all of which can be said to be based on the equity principle:

- the 'demand/utilisation' criterion;
- the 'health situation' criterion;

- the 'coverage by health services' criterion.

The demand/utilisation criterion is based on the principle that every person, throughout the country, should have the same opportunity of utilising the health services. This criterion is based on the application of utilisation rates, by sex and age groups, at national level, and then applied at district level in order to estimate, according to an equity principle, the potential demand foreseen at that level.

The health situation criterion is also applied on an equity basis with a positive (or negative) discrimination factor: districts with a worse health situation will receive a larger allocation of the available total health care resources. The population, in each district, is weighted in respect of a number of health situation indicators: the main age groups; infant mortality rate; specific mortality 1-4 years old, and, SMRs for those aged 5-64 years.

The coverage by health services criterion also adopts an equity principle, and aims to attain the same level of coverage of the risk groups, at the district level. This last criterion is the one that may be considered most original, when compared with the methodology followed in the United Kingdom in the resource allocation of health expenditure on hospital and community services. It is based on the principle of the human capital approach, and recognises that interventions which have as an objective a better level of health may, and should, take place where appropriate outside the health sector. These could come from the income area, the education or the housing area if they can be demonstrated to have an important impact on the level of health of the population.

The human capital approach

It is worth considering the Human Capital approach in more detail as a basis for ensuring greater equity in the allocation of public sector resources to health. It was Grossman (1972) who was one of the first economists to call attention to the fact that health can be likened to a stock, which depreciates over time and which can be increased through investment. Based on Grossman's work, Maynard (1981) described a model of the production of health (Figure 1), thus illustrating the relationship that exists between the inputs which affect health (among which health care is but one aspect) and the resultant outputs.

Le Grand (1982) also argues that it is useful to see health as a capital stock, which depreciates due to the natural process through getting old and, sometimes, also due to unavoidable disease. However, individuals

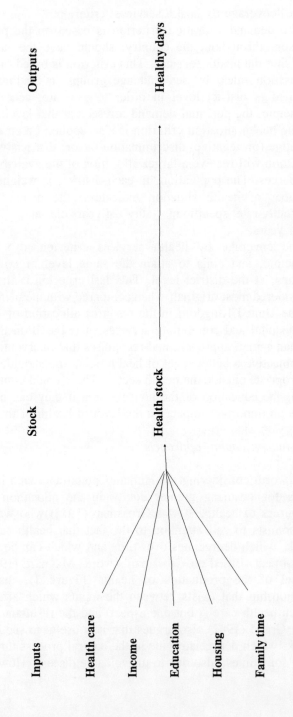

Figure 1: The production of health

Inputs

Health care
Income
Education
Housing
Family time

Stock

Health stock

Outputs

Healthy days

Source: Maynard (1981)

44

can also affect the depreciation process by their own behaviour; investing in health promotion activities (for example, embarking upon regular exercise or receiving adequate medical treatment) which will improve their health stock. They also can increase the depreciation rate through activities which use up their health stock, such as smoking or exposure to unhealthy working conditions.

Ironically, an important part of both public and private health expenditure is used to treat and cure illnesses due to human behaviour resulting in the depreciation of their health capital stock, For instance, Maynard (1985) refers to smoking habits in the United Kingdom, which are probably responsible for 15 to 20 per cent of the total number of deaths per year, and constitute the highest proportion of avoidable deaths in Europe. According to the same author, alcohol consumption has also made an important contribution to premature deaths especially in the last two decades, and this number is increasing. Dearden (1985) refers to the health effects of road traffic accidents that are associated largely with life style, and only to a lesser extent by the road situation and car design. Schwefel (1985) also draws attention to the fact that a country's (or region's) lack of economic stability - as recorded through unemployment - produces premature deaths and morbidity.

This brief review of some of the evidence underlines the need for a multisectoral strategy to the improvement of the health stock of capital.

Conflicts between equity and efficiency principles

Although this is not the main focus of concern in this discussion, it is important to have an overview of the existing conflicts between equity and efficiency principles.

Mooney (1983) makes the distinction between horizontal equity (equal treatment of equals) and vertical equity (differentiation of care according to need) and its conflict with efficiency. Equal treatment of people with equal needs improves equity, which means that horizontal equity goes together with efficiency. It is vertical equity, the unequal treatment of people with different needs, that conflicts with efficiency and this is where a choice will have to be made between the relative weight to be given to an efficiency objective and to an equity objective.

In fact, as Buxton and Klein (1978) noted, resource productivity depends, among other factors, on economies or diseconomies of scale:

> If areas are to provide a comprehensive service for their
> residents, some of the smaller areas are likely to suffer

from inefficient utilisation of more specialist resources. At the other extreme, certain of the larger areas may suffer from diseconomies of scale, perhaps in terms of more difficult and expensive management control (p 16).

However, it can be argued that this conflict between equity and efficiency objectives may not always exist. Sometimes it can happen that promoting equity results, at the same time, in improved efficiency.

Indicators of resource allocation and monitoring

Against this theoretical background the individual studies in this sub-project group have explored the development and application of indicators which could assist in the decision-making processes for resource allocation. The countries and districts participating in the sub-project were: Azores - Portugal; Bohus - Sweden; Dudley - United Kingdom; and, Jamtland - Sweden. The results of the work are outlined below.

The *Azores* study aimed at reviewing and developing quantitative and qualitative indicators to monitor PHC activities, in order to improve decision making and resource allocation process. The project was based on the fact that health care centre budgets were not influenced by a needs based resource allocation formula. Choosing the most useful indicators for planning and decision making, at local level, which was the aim of the study, was an important step to developing resource allocation methods.

The *Bohus County Council* study aimed at developing and introducing a method to monitor primary health care more effectively. This project was based on an existing resource allocation methodology, which had equity as a guiding principle, as it attempted to reallocate resources according to need.

The project sought to assess what the effects are of the relative lack of resources in certain areas. The project was concerned with monitoring in order to try to increase efficiency to reach the goals as fully as possible. An increase of accuracy in statistical reporting and intensive debate of the measurements presently in use today were positive features of the project.

The aim of the *Dudley Health Authority* project was to evaluate the change in provision of long-term care from an institutional setting to small, locally-based nursing homes supported by PHC services, and development of indicators for planning and monitoring the new pattern of service for this client group.

The project , based on the efficiency principle, arrived at the conclusion

46

that comparative costs of nursing homes and long-stay hospital provision indicated that the former was 70% of the cost of in-patient care in a long-stay hospital. Qualitative aspects of being in a nursing home compared to a hospital were made as part of the study. Aspects of privacy, choice (for instance, of waking and getting up routines) regular occupational and leisure activities, and links to the community (for instance, visiting arrangements, opportunities for elderly people to go out) were analysed, the results indicating that these were preferable in the nursing home setting.

The health authority is now reviewing the allocation of resources for the elderly frail within each locality to ensure that needs are related to resource allocation. This would lead to greater emphasis towards the equity principle in determining resource allocation.

The *Jamtland County Council* study on planning and budgeting had the following objectives:

- goal orientated planning and health policy making according to the HFA-strategy;
- need-based budgeting
- monitoring what has been carried out; how it has been carried out; quality measures and costs.
- local democracy and community participation.

The project had an explicit objective of developing a new allocating process of need-based budgeting. At the same time the project, which is wider in scope, sought to achieve greater efficiency through better monitoring.

Conclusion

The common feature of this sub-project was the development and use of indicators as tools for resource allocation and monitoring at both the operational and planning level in participating districts. In Table 5 the individual studies are categorized into indicators for resource allocation, related to equity, and for monitoring, related to efficiency.

Several of the projects propose indicators in order to achieve an equality of input for equal need, that means that they have an equity principle in mind. Others, like the Dudley Health Authority in seeking a balance between community and institutional care for the dependent elderly, propose indicators for monitoring and compare alternative forms

Table 5

Project comparison of indicators for allocation and monitoring

Projects	Indicators for allocation	Indicators for monitoring
1.1 AZORES - PORTUGAL		
Review and development of quantity indicators to monitor PHC activities in order to improve decision making and resource allocation processes.	7 indicators have been selected after 3 Delphi panels having been applied to 5 pre-selected health centres.	
1.2 BOHUS - SWEDEN		
Monitoring of primary health care	The allocation of resources to PHC boards based on a comparison between population need and available resources. The proxy indicators of need are population utilisation of each group of services (GP services, care of the elderly, prevention and so on.) The estimated relative need for the population in each group of service is weighted according to the group % of total cost.	number of visits (GPs and other healthcare workers separately) per inhabitant; number of inpatient days in nursing homes; umber of admissions to these homes; number of patients in home care of the elderly; costs per inhabitant for each service.

Table 5

Project comparison of indicators for allocation and monitoring (continued)

Projects	*Indicators for allocation*	*Indicators for monitoring*
1.3 DUDLEY - UNITED KINGDOM		
Care of frail elderly in community based nursing homes supported by primary health care teams as alternative to long-stay hospital care provision.		% of elderly with a single bedroom; % of elderly who share a bedroom; % of elderly who had choice about daily routines; % of elderly who had regular occupational and leisure activities; % of elderly who were visited by friends; % of elderly who were visited by their relatives or friends.

Table 5

Project comparison of indicators for allocation and monitoring (continued)

Projects	Indicators for allocation	Indicators for monitoring
1.4 JAMTLAND - SWEDEN		
Planning and budgeting Monitoring of primary health care	The allocation of resources is according to need-based budgeting. Consumption is used instead of needs as a practical approximation. The total PHC budget to different activities and to each district. The budget is based on the expected consumption from different age groups of the following activities: medical care (days in-patient; visits) psychiatric care (days in-patient, visits), nursing homes (days in-patient), GPs visits, district nurse visits.	Physicians per 1000 population: Waiting list for specified diagnoses/treatment; patients in hospital; care waiting for discharge; Complications after surgical treatment; % of population with travel time exceeding 20 minutes to GP during working hours; % of patients treated at each level of care; Number of personnel to each patient within the home care for the elderly; Number of terminal care patients who have died in their homes; Number of population getting pensions before 60; Number of patients satisfied with their visit to PHC centre; Rate of vaccination; Rate of readmissions to psychiatric care; Number of parents support groups; Relation between acute/planned admissions to hospital; Number of ambulance transports to PHC centre/hospital; Number of nursing homes used for medical care.

of care, based on an efficiency principle. Based on the work undertaken, the following important points emerge:

*   Equity of inputs per capita for equal need should always be the basis for resource allocation in PHC services;

*   Quantity indicators should be used to indicate the level of coverage of different age groups based on an evaluation of need;

    Quality indicators should allow improvements to be made in the level of need satisfaction already attained;

*   Performance indicators should never influence negatively the resource allocation to population groups but might well influence allocation to providers of care or services;

*   Economic evaluation is always based on a technical efficiency principle and should be used in the comparison of alternatives of care, but not as a basis for resource allocation.

In designing indicators and making them acceptable we would conclude, as for example in the Azores report, that the use of methodology which allows local people to participate in the design of the information system is essential.

4 Community participation and skills development

Marjorie Gott

Introduction

This chapter addresses a range of issues designed to facilitate tipping the balance in health care by opening up decision making, re-orientating professional practice and the development and use of 'education for health' strategies by health professionals. Underpinning all the collaborative projects discussed was the intention to reduce inequity in experiences and expectations of health care, to make services more responsive to local needs, and to make best use of resources, be they fiscal, physical and/or human.

Matching health and welfare provision with the needs of the community is problematic. It is however essential, in a changing society, to ensure the sensitivity of services to local needs, especially when resources are static, or in relative decline. In order to develop and maximise the impact of these services in PHC a well functioning form of participation with the community is a pre-requisite.

In an earlier paper (Godinho, 1990) three different change structures for Tipping The Balance Towards Primary Health Care were identified. These were described as restructuring, re-education and facilitation. This discussion is concerned with issues of re-education and facilitation. It explores facilitative strategies for community participation, collaboration between health care workers and clients, service reorientations, and the necessary re-education of health professionals in order that they can promote common health messages to the populations with whom they work.

In addition to requiring new knowledge to undertake health promotion work, workers are required to develop a range of skills. These include interactive skills, teaching skills, teamwork skills and skills in the management of change. This group of skills is commonly known as health promotion skills.

As mentioned in chapter one, PHC structures, roles and relationships differ between countries, and failure to acknowledge this at the outset would render what follows open to misinterpretation. The fact that organisation of PHC varies widely between 'developed' countries has been noted by WHO (1986).

> In some countries well coordinated teams form the established and recognised first point of contact with the official health system. In others, access to health care may be through general practitioners, specialists or nurses, all working alone. In many countries, people belonging to particular social groups or living in a particular geographical areas are still without good access to primary health care services are less generally available than curative services(p.47).

In addition to differences in levels of, and access to, PHC services between countries, there are also differences of interpretation. Vuori (1984) has remarked on the distinction between primary *health* care, and primary *medical* care:

> The claim that primary medical care is identical with primary health care is particularly dear to those health authorities and professionals who want to give the impression of being all for primary health care but who in fact are either opposed to it, or have not quite understood what it means (p.221).

The difficulty in getting mutual understanding about the role and remit of PHC was recognised at the outset of the TTB project and it was universally agreed that the operational concept of PHC that participants would work with would be based on the Alma Ata Declaration. Four ways of interpreting PHC were identified:

*   As a philosophy, reinforcing the notions of justice and equity;
*   As a principle, incorporating the notion of free, open, and relevant access to all who need it;
*   As the first point of health care contact;
*   As a set of activities concerned with disease prevention and treatment, rehabilitation and health promotion.

In adopting the above as the definition of PHC with which the overall project would work, participants were mindful of the need for a 'living' definition; one that could be used in a diverse range of action research projects. They were also aware that an operational definition was long overdue. These understandings underpin the TTB Project as a whole, and are evident in the projects that will be discussed in this section. Legitimacy for the adoption of the working definition and the type of research activity engaged in the TTB project is found in the WHO HFA Evaluation Report (1986):

> ... a great deal of thought had been given to defining the functions and responsibilities of the health care sector, but less attention has been paid to implementing the changes called for and to integrating the activities of primary, secondary and tertiary levels into a coherent whole (p.47).

This sub-project is divided into specific areas which are united by a common core. The common objectives are to:

* explore and enhance different ways and methods of involving local communities in decisions about the provision of PHC;

* analyse and develop different methods of improving PHC sensitivity to local needs and/or changing patterns of disease;

* establish methods of promoting healthier lifestyles in the community;

* improve intersectoral collaborative working;

* reorient health care from the secondary and tertiary care sector to the primary care sector;

* improve the health promotion skills of health practitioners.

The projects reported in this paper address these common objectives.

Tipping the balance: community participation and skills development

The projects analysed in this chapter are diverse in their scope, and need to be interpreted in terms of the quite different contexts (geographical and practice) from which they are drawn. Nonetheless, when one looks at the studies in their entirety, common problems, issues, strategies and solutions are fairly evident. There are eleven studies in the sub-project

54

drawn from Eastern Health Board - Ireland; Viseu - Portugal; Valencia - Spain; Alvsberg, Blenkinge, Jamtland - Sweden; Dudley, North Staffordshire, West Lambeth - United Kingdom. They fall naturally into the following three action areas: community participation, prevention and health promotion; and, reorientation to PHC.

Community participation

There are three projects in this category, two in the United Kingdom (North Staffordshire and West Lambeth) and one in Sweden (Jamtland). The underlying premise for this group of interventions was: local participation will assist statutory bodies to develop and improve services more effectively by creating partnership with the community and its resources. For partnership to occur, structures for dialogue and action needed to be created. These needed to be both formal and informal. As Siler Wells (1988) has noted, strengthening community health means strengthening the community. She advocates doing this by creating a supportive policy focus; mobilising political and community will; supporting new partnerships; and co-action.

These strategies were deployed by the teams working on this initiative. But in order to use them they had to think very hard about the meaning of 'community'. Many writers contend that there is not such thing as the 'community'; it being a neat and cosy aberration in the heads of politicians, planners and practitioners. It is conceptually neat, but non existent in real life; 'communities' being made up of a rich diversity of groups and interests. What is common to such groups however is geographical location; they live in neighbourhoods. These can be identified by both physical characteristics (for example number, type, and state of buildings for public use), and by their general ethos or spirit (run down or buzzing with activity).

Neighbourhoods can be defined as a limited area identified as such by people living there with reference to common residence, common interest, and mutual benefit and obligation. The empirical value of using neighbourhoods as discrete units for service delivery and analysis has been described by Kivell *et al* (1990).

The purpose for the introduction of Neighbourhood Forums in *North Staffordshire* was equity in local health service decision-making by involving consumers, as well as providers, in decision-making arenas. The creation of forums on their own was seen as having little potential for success if not supported by intra and inter-organisational changes. These included decentralisation of management structures, decentralisation of budgetary control, and development of effective information systems. These systems were put in place. The findings show that Neighbourhood Forums were successfully achieving their aims of increasing local involvement and partnership in health related decision-making, and of addressing those needs which communities themselves have identified. As a result of this initiative new services are being provided, and better use being made of community resources (physical and human). These are now viewed as being used more flexibly and more creatively.

The survey conducted by the *West Lambeth Patch* project concluded that 'lay' participation was essential in decisions affecting health in the community, not only to ensure that provision was appropriate, but also because the views of the community differ so widely from those of the health professionals responsible for resources and service delivery. Findings indicated that people's needs were not just for efficient health services; the advancement of health was not a matter for health services alone, collaboration was necessary. Many management groups were invisible to health service providers and attitudes to health and health services were correspondingly poor. Perception of factors affecting health ranged widely between the health professions and the community they served.

Recommendations included the need for decentralised structures to allow for lay participation, empowerment through resourcing the community's involvement, and effective inter-sectoral collaboration. Factors affecting health, especially in the inner-city, go far beyond the capacity of the health services in isolation to deliver.

The objective of the *Jamtland* study was to evaluate the protocolled activity of eight locally appointed political boards. Hypothetically there would be expected to be a shift from budget dominated work to more health strategic work aiming at community responsiveness, local flexibility and reorientation. Results showed that the majority of the protocolled decisions were purely administrative. It was found that local boards had difficulty in delegating forums and administrative work, though a positive trend towards delegation was noted. No evident evolution was seen towards more health promoting activities or PHC strategy.

Criteria for measuring participation in PHC have been developed by an international group of experts working for both WHO and UNICEF (Rifkin *et al* 1988; Bichmann *et al* 1989). To date 200 case studies in participation have been reviewed by them and five key factors identified: needs assessment; leadership; organisation; resource mobilisation; and, management.

These five 'participation' criteria were evident in each of the identified sub-projects, with differing degrees of strength. Participation helps make PHC more responsive to 'bottom up'priorities and needs. When it works it enables people to be more confident in their dealings with professionals. For people to reach this stage they must be educated and informed about the health care system, and their own rights, responsibilities and powers. This calls for new attitudes on the part of all involved; people and professionals alike. Reorientation of professional attitudes and practices is discussed in the following section.

Prevention and health promotion

There were four projects under this umbrella heading from Sweden (two in Blekinge) and United Kingdom (Dudley and North Staffordshire). Whilst all are concerned with health promotion activities, some points of focus were different. Two, *Blekinge and Dudley*, were concerned with developing and extending the preventive skills of PHC professionals. Another study, also from *Blekinge*, took reduction of coronary heart disease as its aim, but adopted quite different strategies, using non-professionals to give teaching to local groups in the community. The other project, *North Staffordshire*, focused upon reducing inequality in the perinatal mortality rates of health districts.

In the previous section the discussion identified the need for professionals, as well as the public, to develop new attitudes for health work. Earlier in the chapter the view that PHC professionals may not value preventive activities was advanced (Vuori, 1984). There is an extensive literature to support this assertion (Gott 1986; Calnan 1986; and Green 1987). In a study of health promotion and education training needs Spratley and Gott (1988) found that:

> Many practising doctors and nurses will need support in
> developing skills for health promotion work since their
> basic training has not tended to concentrate on
> interpersonal skills, teaching skills and shared health
> care planning(p.12).

In recent years there has been a growing recognition that many PHC workers need and want to develop their health promotion skills. Two major ways of doing this are through in service continuing education, and by the provision of a facilitator to PHC teams. One of the most popular forms of continuing education is distance learning in which PHC members study together, where and when they like, about a chosen health issue. A good example of this is the Open University teaching package for PHC workers: 'Coronary Heart Disease: Reducing the risk'. This is often used in conjunction with a facilitator. A facilitator specialises in preventative medicine, management of change and skills training. He/she acts as an adviser, motivator and support person to teams who wish to develop their preventive work. *Dudley* used such a facilitator to work with its teams, and, in particular, to train nurses to work in different ways.

The major health problem in the developed countries is coronary heart disease. Enormous financial and human resources are being devoted to its reduction. Two general approaches are evident: the mass population approach and the high risk approach. The mass population approach involves giving 'stay low' (reduce unhealthy behaviour) messages to the population at large; the high risk approach involves opportunistic finding of CHD risks in people who attend health centres, for whatever reason. It is the latter approach which was the prominent feature of two of the sub-project studies: Blenkinge and Dudley. Table 6 summarises the key features of each approach.

Coronary Heart Disease (CHD) is the dominate cause of death in Sweden. During the last few years it has been fully recognized in *Blekinge* that prevention of ischemic heart disease demands a community strategy in combination with a medical one. Therefore, one of the *Blekinge* Projects was concentrated on primary prevention of cardiac and arterial disease by opportunistic screening in a PHC district. The study indicated the feasibility of using multiple cardiovascular risk factor intervention in PHC with resources presently used for hypertension management. The results also indicated that a substantial proportion of the population at risk will be detected.

In this programme, screening for hypercholesteroleamia was integrated with regular case finding for hypertension which is an established component of general practice. No facilitator was used, as it was seen as essential that PHC nurses work together with general practitioners (GPs) as a normal part of their preventive programme which had its basis in regular care, as this was a way of keeping the general profile of work. All the necessary motivation, training, education and management for facilitation of this opportunistic CHD prevention programme occurred collaboratively, and was integrated in the every day work of doctors and nurses. However nurses took on the role of educator for self-care.

58

Table 6
Approaches for reducing coronary heart disease

High risk approach	*Population approach*
* Focuses on high risk individual who have most to gain from changing	* Requires everyone to change a little. But little motivation (gain) can be offered
* Relatively little effect on mass disease, i.e. health of the nation	* More effective against mass disease, i.e. improving health of the nation
* Danger of 'victim blaming' by identifying high risk 'deviant'	* Since most people could reduce their risks it becomes a generally desirable activity with less risk of 'victim blaming'
* Difficult for individuals to change when social and economic pressures may oppose change	* Promotes social and economic changes making it easier for the individual to change
* Only high risk individuals are worried, though some unnecessarily	* Danger that the whole community becomes anxious/ obsessed avoiding heart disease
* Does not encourage individuals to keep their risks low. Can often give false reassurance if bordering on more than one factor	* Overall emphasis on 'staying low' - keeping risk factors down
* Traditional medical model approach appeals to PHC team	* Health promotion approach, especially on need for socio-economic change, less familiar to PHC team
* Treats individuals as 'patient'; doctor/nurse use familiar skills	* Models relationship as 'partners for health'; requires unfamiliar health educator skills

Source: *Coronary Heart Disease: Reducing the Risk, 1987: 575*

The coronary heart disease rate for *Dudley* is above the United Kingdom national average. The *Dudley* project team decided that it would systematically screen people aged between 30-65 years for risk factors for heart disease and encourage the development of a healthy lifestyle. Results showed that advising patients individually at screening sessions was more effective than attempting to get them to attend groups. It was believed that this was because the population did not see group education as part of their culture and were particularly resistant to 'quit smoking' groups as they saw smoking as helping them to cope (this finding is in line with empirical work from elsewhere). Dietary advice was much more successful: PHC teams reported a significant fall in cholesterol levels following dietary advice.

It was noted above that there are distinctions between the high risk approach to CHD, and the mass population approach. Although there are some who remain formally wedded to the idea of using just one of these approaches, the general, and growing, consensus is that both approaches are necessary (Open University, 1987). *Blekinge* has worked in such a way, using a high risk approach and also a mass population approach (see table 6).

The *Blekinge* County Council had another project aimed at health promotion through a discussion among the general public. Co-operation between the County Council and the County Study Association led to the start of study circles in all municipalities and in local study associations. Employees in the hospitals and PHC had the opportunity to join study circles during working-time in order to exchange experiences. The County Council had taken an important step in line with WHO principles to renew the methods for better public health. Basic facts and proposals for health-political discussions have been presented. The general public was deeply interested in health matters and many persons were ready to take part in preventive actions and improving public health.

The County Council had decided to revise the study-material and to present an up-dated version during 1991. New study circles also started, especially these occurring in co-operation with a number of trade unions. It was assumed that the discussions about new diseases, about health and social structures and about health and life-styles would increase the awareness among the general public of the risk factors for ischemic heart disease and therefore promote healthier lifestyles.

Underpinning the *North Staffordshire* Health Authority project to reduce perinatal mortality was the awareness that health experiences and expectations are influenced by inequalities in the social conditions and situations in which people find themselves. The starkest example of social inequality is premature (avoidable) death. Farrent and Taft (1988) believe that certain kinds of policy create unhealthy and unequal social climates. They note however that even the poorest districts can work to reduce inequality. In discussing their experiences with a poor inner London district they found:

> the main health enhancing aspects of the districts were seen as living and residing in the people working there - specifically the resourcefulness of a lively multi-racial community, an active voluntary sector, and socially aware and committed field workers (p. 295).

They go on to note that innovative practice often arises in such circumstances.

The *North Staffordshire* project is a case in point. The aim of the project was to influence a reduction in perinatal mortality by promoting preconceptual care in the community. Level of knowledge about both healthy lifestyles and specific preconceptual care information was tested in a mixed group of professionals in two districts. A high knowledge about healthy lifestyles was found (however this is not necessarily transferable into teaching or client behaviour). Additional teaching was provided in training sessions and an information pack containing health education literature was distributed.

Group members identified priority action areas for the population: reduction of smoking, increased exercise activity, improvement of parenting skills, provision of health promotion sessions in the school and workplace. Staff recognised that life style education, though important, was likely to be ineffective on its own. People needed opportunities to change, as well as information. Recognising this, staff have designed interventions that also seek to influence contexts (school, workplace). By doing this, and also by acting as role models (exercise initiative) it was hoped that behaviour change would be supported.

Reorientation to primary health care

Whilst all the TTB projects have this intention in general, some projects had taken it as their specific focus for intervention. These were Alvsborg (Sweden), Eastern Health Board (Ireland), Valencia (Spain), Viseu (Portugal), and West Lambeth (United Kingdom).

The *Alvsborg* project was concerned with improving health care communication especially between trained nurses and patients. The working assumption was that the development of guidelines applicable to both PHC and hospitals would strengthen patients and community confidence in PHC. A noteworthy feature of this initiative was the extension of the role of the nurse as a keyworker in PHC, which highlights a growing trend in the development of this type of nursing role. Not only was it more efficient, it was more cost effective, and it was also well accepted by patients.

More PHC doctors and nurses are now working in partnership to develop and use protocols for management of patient symptoms. Most frequently this is in hypertension management (Fullard, 1987, Farquar and Bowling, 1990). This strategy is proving so successful that management of other common ailments (asthma, diabetes) is now also being initially undertaken by nurses working in PHC settings.

Some PHC units have gone further than this and employed and trained nurse practitioners. Stillwell is a Nurse Practitioner in the United Kingdom. Like the Alvsborg nurses, she has had extra training for this role. She consults in a similar pattern to doctors, during surgery hours, the patients having a choice of whom they wish to see. Consultation times with patients are longer (20 minutes as opposed to 6), and she uses agreed protocols for management of common problems. Patients see her role as: 'having a responsibility for encouraging long-term health measures such as stopping smoking, losing weight or having a smear test' for cervical cancer. (Stillwell *et al*, 1987:156). This type of role is similar to that undertaken by practice nurses in the Dudley project aimed at reducing CHD.

Another study which uses nurses in an innovative way was the *Valencia* project which used midwives in PHC to help reduce inequity in childbirth experiences. An explicit aim was to promote both the public health system and the (new) PHC model. The project analysed motivation to use, and satisfaction with, public versus private prenatal services. It seems that the new model was more accessible physically than the traditional model for the pregnant women. This possibly only reflects the fact that the new model has been installed geographically in the most densely populated areas. This was a logical priority when planning services.

The new PHC model was effective at promoting the use of prenatal care services among the exposed population. However, when the socio-economic level component was added, as a necessary determinant, the new model was not more accessible for women of middle-low socio-economic level. The use of prenatal care by these women was significantly lower. The prenatal care offered by the new model to the public sector was used more intensively by women from the middle-high sector.

The remaining two projects in this group also demonstrated reorientation of health care towards the PHC sector. The *Viseu* project was concerned with improving GPs work on mental health care, as well as improving cooperation between PHC and secondary care (mental health clinic).

The team recognised that the quality of mental health medical referral was poor and so special training was provided for GPs to improve the quantity and quality of their work on mental health. A protocol of good practice was developed and, on later evaluation of its use, it was found that both quantity and quality of referral by GPs to specialists had improved. In the context of intrasectoral cooperation and integration of PHC and mental health care, the information and training strategy followed proved relevant.

The *West Lambeth* project involved the provision of a small 20 bedded short-stay and day-care Community Centre, to both extend PHC services and meet care needs caused by the closure of an existing hospital. The aim was to keep people who were in need of professional health care in the community and to provide a medical and nursing service that was locally based, informal and personal in its approach, with the onus on the whole person in their family and social environment. The Centre was managed by a multi-disciplinary local team including health and welfare professionals and community members. An especially notable feature of the initiative was the decision, at an early stage to appoint a community link worker to help the community identify its health needs and to learn about, use, and shape the Centre (although this proved an extremely successful initiative, when funds ran out, the worker was not re-appointed).

An evaluation study was carried out after three years of the Centres existence. Findings indicate that the Centre clearly was seen as part of the community and there was evidence of ownership of its values and purpose (the creation of the Centre had been supported by a strong local community action movement). It was strongly felt however that as communities are diverse, the needs of some groups might have gone unrecognised. The project Action group was very aware of this dilemma and had identified a number of strategies for increasing community involvement, but due to lack of funds, were unable to implement them.

Discussion and conclusion

In reviewing these studies certain things stand out in sharp relief. The first of these is their universality. It is evident that, whatever the country, whatever the initiative, certain common principles exist. These are:

* *Community responsiveness* in which genuine attempts have been made to work from the bottom up to seek to identify what kind of a service it is that people want and how, or even whether, this fits with what has traditionally been provided by health professionals.

* *Collaboration* has been demonstrated in all of the projects discussed. In some instances the emphasis has been on improved collaboration between different professionals, in others between professionals and clients and in some, better multiple collaborations between all interested parties. Collaboration occasionally has involved some restructuring of services, and, often skill development so that better teamwork could occur.

* *Effectiveness* - The WHO declaration on Primary Health Care emphasises the issue of effectiveness in locating services within PHC. These projects have also sought to demonstrate, given a growing acceptance that factors effecting health are not meliorated by hospital care, why PHC is a more effective strategy for policy makers.

* *Teamwork* is a more active form of collaboration in which participants work intensively together to create, manage and evaluate their performance in relation to a particular initiative. A concrete example to teamwork, demonstrated by both the Dudley and Alvsborg projects, was the joint production of protocols to manage ill health.

* *Reorientation* in philosophy, practice, and service location also has been described. Working with broader (social) notions of health, coalitions of people have come together to change aspects of service delivery, provide new services and work with the hospital sector to reduce length of stay in acute settings.

* *Inequality* with regard to health experiences and expectations characterised many of the populations in the whole Tipping The Balance Project. In particular disparities have been noted in rates for coronary heart disease and perinatal mortality. There exists, in all of the countries participating in the project , an underclass who

experience significantly higher levels of mortality and morbidity than the general population. It has been the intention of project workers to find practical, relevant and locally sensitive ways to seek to reduce inequality in the mortality and morbidity rates of the populations with whom they work. The Valencia project is a good example of this kind of initiative.

*   *Equity* means fairness of service distribution. Recognising that the most disadvantaged , for a variety of reasons, make least use of statutory health services - and so remain in a 'Catch 22' situation as regards poor health, workers have gone into community settings and begun to work with networks that residents themselves have generated. In both North Staffordshire, and West Lambeth there has been genuine attempt to identify, and work with, all sectors of the community.

*   *Social justice* is the notion that unites the above concepts and has been one of the guiding principles of the Tipping The Balance Project. It recognises the value of concepts such as the 'empowerment' and 'participation' of individuals, but also acknowledges the role that society plays in shaping opportunities for individual behaviour change.

All the efforts documented in this chapter clearly indicate that the sub-project teams are making a major contribution towards social justice in health care. In addition to reviewing principles, there are other important conclusions that can be drawn which particularly are action-orientated. These are:

*   Participation allows for 'bottom up' service development, and is fundamental to reorientation;

*   For reorientation and participation to occur, staff attitudes and practices need to change;

*   Change will allow for the development of new roles, including that of key workers, who will be a point of first PHC contact (e.g. facilitator);

*   These changes require new PHC management structures and the development of common action protocols for managing health risks

and lifestyle behaviour changes;

*   To be successful these initiatives must not occur in isolation, collaborative interventions require changed structures and management of resources; part of the jigsaw in the HFA 2000 Picture, part of the agenda is consensus building for successful management of change.

It is strongly recommend that the philosophies, strategies and interventions discussed in this chapter are used in Primary Health Care basic and post-basic education and that practitioners from different professional groups be encouraged to model the Health For All principles of teamworking and common problem solving that have been demonstrated by the Tipping the Balance Project.

5 Tipping the balance towards primary health care: Practice, training and research

Joana Godinho and Marjorie Gott

Introduction

The Project has been succeeded in its overall objective of contributing to the process of 'tipping the balance' towards Primary Health Care, through not only empowerment of services at the first level, but also through a bottom-up approach which sought to return health and development initiative to the end users; individuals living in communities. The Project has also contributed to the integration of health research and practice at the European level, one of the main aims of the action programmes of the Commission of the European Communities.

Besides these general goals, the Tipping The Balance Project also sought to achieve four additional objectives: to describe and demonstrate PHC in action; to provide models and mechanisms that can be seen to work at the local/district level; to promote locally-based, locally sensitive research; and, to create an European network for PHC research and practice. Three out of the four specific objectives of the Project were achieved. However, the Project was only partially successful with regard to the second objective.

What follows is an analysis of the outcomes of the Project in light of both the general goals and the specific ones. The discussion then turns to the Project achievements and results. This is followed by the main conclusions for each area of work (decentralisation, indicators, community participation and skills development) and for the whole Project. It ends with recommendations for practice, training and research on Primary Health Care.

Review of project objectives

Objective 1 -To provide a description of current levels of organisation

and management of local/district-based primary health care services and provide a set of common definitions about PHC.

This objective has been achieved. A picture of Primary Health Care is provided, based on twenty one case-studies developed in fifteen districts of seven European countries. The case studies and the analyses of the three main sub-project areas provide a detailed portrait. Definitions of key-PHC concepts were also agreed and are reviewed in this report.

It is clear that the discussion does not provide a complete picture of the European first level of health care: it was not intended to do this. Participant countries and districts have developed PHC services to differing degrees, using different structures and approaches, but within the same public-oriented framework. For this reason descriptions provided are useful, not only to countries and districts with similar systems, but as points of comparison for others.

Objective 2 - To clarify and evaluate, according to their stage of development, some potentially relevant and effective organisation models and mechanisms that can contribute to 'tipping the balance' towards improved provision of primary health care, by conducting experimental studies in three linked key areas;

(a)   decentralisation of primary health care;
(b)   indicators for resource allocation and monitoring in PHC;
(c)   community participation and skills for PHC workers.

This objective was partly achieved. Case-studies were undertaken in the three linked areas, and some relevant organisational models and mechanisms were identified. However, whereas the impact of these models and mechanisms over health services processes and outputs is clear in some cases, it is not at all clear in others. For example, whilst it has been possible to state that decentralisation is occurring in all health services involved, and to characterise the stage of decentralisation for the sub-project participant districts, there is some ambiguity surrounding the true extent of decentralisation that has taken place. This may be partly explained by the following:

*   the fact that projects were at different stages of development;

*   different mechanisms and structures in different countries offer different opportunities;

68

* the 'unfreezing' stage of social change affecting health services that was highlighted in the North Staffordshire case-study on local participation (Gott and Warren, 1990). Studies from Orebro, Jamtlands, and West Lambeth also refer to this and its consequences whereby further action/research becomes either impossible or irrelevant because of change in policies (due to a change in direction, or lack of resources). The innovation then becomes 'frozen'.

In spite of these problems, the Project still demonstrates that there are some effective models and mechanisms that can contribute to 'tipping the balance' towards PHC. These include devolution as a decentralisation strategy, employment of a facilitator as a linchpin for PHC; and, shifts in secondary/primary health care roles and responsibilities to enable services to be both more efficient and more responsive (see in particular the Alvsborg and Dudley case studies in Part II).

Objective 3 - To promote the development of locally-based research, by studying locally relevant issues with adequate scientific support.

This objective was almost completely achieved. Local relevant issues for action-research were identified by participants, through a pedagogic consultation process. A significant omission however is that, for a Project that so strongly advocates a 'bottom-up' approach to health problems, representatives of communities were sometimes not explicitly engaged in the problem identification process. This omission should be corrected in any further action oriented projects aimed at Tipping The Balance Towards Primary Health Care.

Locally-based research took place and, in certain cases, continues far beyond the time frame of the Project (for example, in the Dudley and Blekinge related work). In the great majority of the cases, research was successfully completed, with 'mortality' for participation being kept to a minimum. It is worth making the point here however that some districts/countries have had more difficulty than others in participating in such an international activity, because of lack of resources or skills, and limited access to adequate scientific support to carry out action-research successfully. Therefore, it is recommended that in the future special attention and support be given to overcoming such obstacles.

Adequate scientific support was provided by over a half a dozen academic institutions and by at least a dozen individual academic researchers, either by working at the case-study, sub-project or at the project level. In addition, technical assistance was provided by WHO/Europe and by the EC appointed 'chef-de-file'. The successful cooperation between the 'industry' (health services, in this case), academic institutions (schools of public health and universities), and international organisations (WHO and EC), is one of the most significant achievements of this Project.

Objective 4 - To create an European network of district-based researchers, who will act beyond the time frame of the Project.

This objective was completely achieved. Despite many cultural, organisational and managerial problems, a network of about 50 district-based health researchers has been created. The network has had remarkably low 'mortality', and now has over five years experience of local, district, country and European common work. This is no mean achievement. The Project success is well documented in the quality of the case-studies presented in Part II of this volume.

An additional benefit is that many links were established between teams and institutions within and between countries, and they will persist and be effective beyond the time frame of the Project.

The formal products of the Project are an edition of the European Journal of Public Health featuring a Summary of the Project, this book and a new proposal for a Concerted Action. In this proposal, new lines of work are to be explored, based on the experience already gained, and new teams will be involved, as some initial ones withdraw. However, other linkages and cooperative work is being pursued, as illustrated by the United Kingdom/Sweden cooperation on the local participation study and action towards decreasing cardio-vascular disease, and by linkages between health services and academic institutions from different countries (for example, Spain/United Kingdom/Yugoslavia) to improve services, training and research on PHC.

Project results

The case-studies are the basis of the Project, providing the core results, and the previous chapters carefully analysed them and drew some conclusions. Based on the case-studies and the preceding discussion, the results and draw general conclusions that apply to the overall Project are now highlighted.

1   Managing decentralisation of primary health care.

The objectives of the sub-project were to assess whether decentralisation of health services is an efficient and effective way of delivering health care and meeting community needs, and to identify similarities between the different systems and assess its significance. Porvoo and the Eastern Health Board studies proposed models for decentralisation with decision-making and budgetary autonomy. The Porvoo approach, which stressed team working and budgetary autonomy, is already being adopted by other districts in Finland, while the Eastern Health Board model is being implemented by the Board in Dublin and surrounding areas.

The Andalucia and North Staffordshire studies propose models for evaluation of decentralisation of PHC that were being used already to analyse the present situation. While the first study concentrated on needs, values and attitudes, accessibility and quality of care, the second related costs with benefits and quality of services. Zadar also carried out an evaluation study, while Orebo carried out and evaluated experiments on further decentralisation. This last study concluded that the experiments had limited impact on efficiency and increased democracy, but local units came out of them much stronger. Moreover, a significant observation arising from this work is that it is not possible to decentralise below a certain level.

As the researchers in Orevo remarked, 'the impact of an organisational change cannot be estimated until after at least 5 years'. Nevertheless while decentralisation of health services and PHC in fact was taking place in the majority of the districts involved, it was notable that a hybrid form was more common rather than clear cut models of decentralisation. Most districts fit in between delegation and devolution, except for Zadar, where the new trend seems to be the opposite, pointing towards increased centralisation. As was pointed out in chapter two, decentralisation does appear to have had a relatively positive impact on workers involved, as well as (were it was possible to evaluate in some cases), a positive impact on provision of care.

2   Indicators for planning and resource allocation in PHC.

The sub-project was concerned primarily with monitoring PHC and resource allocation according to needs, although, in common with the first sub-project, there was some interest in decentralisation of decision-making. The specific objectives were to propose both qualitative and quantitative indicators of PHC that would help in planning and needs-

71

based resource allocation. Interest in monitoring was raised in all districts. Some participating districts developed indicators that included criteria of both equity and efficiency, while others only considered efficiency. None followed the human capital approach that Giraldes and Daley outlined in chapter three.

In its move from hospital to community-based care for the elderly, Dudley improved efficiency, and proposed indicators of success for decentralised care. Bohus explored the idea on an indicator of 'profit', and tried to link monitoring with increased efficiency and achievement of goals based on needs, (and was only partly successful). This district is now proposing decentralisation of information to individual decision makers, to avoid decisions being taken without adequate consideration of the available information. Jamtlands, which has detailed an innovative list of indicators (Table 5), also advised that information be decentralised to local managers.

The list of indicators proposed by these studies for monitoring, planning and budgeting according to needs (Table 5), covers indirect measures of needs (for example, mortality rates, consumption of services, prescriptions, need for home service), and some indicators of outcome (life length and quality of life of the elderly). What must be of especial concern is the lack of proposals concerning health promotion indicators, as it is such an important activity on the framework of PHC, and offers participation both by health services and by society. There are only two districts (Azores and Jamtlands) which tried to develop proposals for disease prevention indicators . It is imperative, therefore, that further work be undertaken on developing indicators for effective health promotion.

3   *Increasing community participation and developing skills for PHC.*

The sub-project sought to identify different ways and methods of involving the communities in PHC decision making, delivery and evaluation, and of increasing PHC sensitivity to local health needs and issues. Another focus was that of developing the health protection and promotion skills of health workers. In most instances workers were trained health professionals, in others (Blekinge) 'lay' workers were involved. It was found that multi-faceted initiatives involving both professional and lay workers, working in partnership, were especially successful.

Concerning the role of local boards, North Staffordshire concluded that while local boards are successful, they needed improvements in attendance and involvement. Jamtlands noted that local boards have difficulty in delegating and that they tended to concentrate more on administrative issues rather than on strategic thinking. West Lambeth observed that in PHC more attention should be given to needs than to spurious measures of 'efficiency'. They also made the point that true (rather than rhetorical) community involvement needed to be resourced, and cited, sadly, the fact that the community linkperson appointed to the project, whilst highly valued and highly necessary to the project's success, was terminated because funds (or commitment?) ran out. This type of short-term financial driven thinking invariably bedevils efforts to tip the balance towards community sensitive PHC.

On intra- and intersectoral-cooperation issues, chapter four noted the importance of the need for common preparation of health professionals and public sector professionals. The evidence from the TTB studies is that different types of workers are keen and willing to work together for the common good, and that they are at their most effective when they do so. It is surely both more sensible and more cost effective to offer common training programmes at entry into the professionals rather than to have to offer special post qualifying courses on teaching people how to work together collaboratively when they have already been practising for a number of years.

The Alvsborg study clearly demonstrated that nurses may be more efficient, cost-effective and have greater acceptability in health promotion work than other health professionals. The Valencia study also found that midwives are preferred to doctors and, although working in the public sector, offer a service as good as private care in maternal and child health. Therefore, this suggests that both the role and skills of nurses and of midwives could and should be enhanced within PHC.

Three of the studies on health promotion and disease prevention activities (two in Blekinge and one in Dudley) showed that both a mass population and a high-risk/opportunistic approach can be appropriate to reducing cardio-vascular disease. Moreover, Blekinge demonstrated that using resources that were allocated to a smaller problem (hypertension) to help solve a bigger one, coronary heart disease, coupled with a high risk approach can have positive benefits.

Not all of the studies reported in sub-project 3 have been completed by the time the project ended; some are in mid-phase (the perinatal mortality study), others will be continuing (neighbourhood forums, CHD risk reduction, public midwives). As projects evolve, shift, develop and grow, participants and communities grow with them. As Hayes *et al* (1990) point out, communities are diverse; there is no 'one [that] fits all solutions'. There are common issues that threaten health however (poverty, low self-esteem, lack of organisation). Many of the case studies have shown how these essentially social justice issues can be tackled through common commitment, goodwill and collaboration.

In summary, the balance definitely has been tipped towards improved and more participatory primary health care. Action research conducted at the local/district level, has had a significant impact on services and, to a lesser extent, on communities and their health needs. From the experience of Tipping The Balance Project, there is a need for re-orientation not only of the health services, but of the attitude of professionals and decision-makers in health and other related sectors, as well as of individuals living in communities. The underlying principles for this statement are that:

*   health is a priceless commodity;

*   health is the shared responsibility of individuals, health services, and communities, not only in what concerns the individual health budget and health future, but in relation to the common good;

*   healthy lives and healthy choices can be facilitated by the health services pursual of decentralisation to the local level (not only geographic; including resources and decision-making);

*   needs and equity should be overriding concerns for information seeking, decision-making, planning and budgeting;

*   partnership must be created between communities and health services, to identify needs and seek ways of addressing them. This can be achieved through different forms of community participation, such as formal participation on local boards, or formal partnerships, as for instance, in 'study' circles.

Project recommendations

The main recommendations of the Project are of relevance to PHC services and professionals operating at all levels, and to international agencies concerned with health care and health care training. They fall into three areas: practice, training and research. Each is now considered in turn.

Primary health care practice: The 'bottom-up' approach that is so important to facilitating participation is recommended. Its success depends on the following requirements:

* decentralisation, not only geographical, but also of decision-making and resource allocation;

* allocation of sufficient physical and financial resources;

* community data banks of information, which are dynamic, and underpin the work of PHC and related services;

* community participation in health-related decision-making and new skills for PHC workers, which will prepare them to engage in working with and training others.

Primary health care training: The case-studies documented in this book are about 'real life'. Therefore, they will be useful for training health and health related professionals, and for encouraging training institutions and networks to use them as examples of what is occurring in PHC, and what works, under what conditions. This recommendation is consistent with that made by WHO (1990) on priorities for continuing education in PHC.

Common training of health and health related professionals, for example, public health doctors, nurses, and managers, health related professionals and social workers is an important lesson from the Project. As is the training of health and health related personnel in new key roles, as facilitators of community participation and health promotion activities, and network managers prepared to engage in intra- and inter-sectoral cooperation. Finally, it is recommended that training includes carrying out action-research activities, which will encourage professionals to evaluate their work and PHC activities.

Primary health care research: The Project pursued the action-research line of work at the district/local level. In the course of undertaking the twenty one different studies, additional areas of work have been identified. There are three important lines of research for PHC which require further exploration:

* *Monitoring the implementation and evaluation of PHC*: including working on and refining indicators that will pay special attention to health needs, health promotion interventions, and their relevance to the health of individuals and communities;

*   *Exploring the utilization of market incentives in PHC*: namely the idea of public competition and of privatisation, and programme and clinical budgeting and their impact on efforts to further tip the balance towards primary health care;

*   *Exploring the community development approach*: namely by studying ways of resourcing community participation, and by developing new roles and relationships in primary health care.

It is argued that though the efforts documented in Part II, and by further development along the lines indicated above, the 'TTB' project will continue to make a significant international contribution towards enabling European health care systems to more fully embrace and deliver the Primary Health Care that their citizens deserve and need.

Part II
COUNTRY CASE STUDIES

Finland

Primary health care

Primary Health Care services in Finland has developed rapidly since 1972 when the Public Health Act was passed. The responsibility to organise PHC services was defined by legislation. Every commune in the country should, either by itself or together with one or more other communes, provide all the necessary PHC services for its population. Thus the country with its 5 million population was divided into approximately 220 health centre districts, each responsible for providing the primary health care services. This includes primary medical care, preventive care, environmental health care, dental care and care of the elderly and chronically ill at health centre hospitals.

The population of a health centre varies from 10,000 to 50,000 the average being approximately 17,500 inhabitants when the 5 largest cities are excluded. Health centres are locally administered by a political board of representatives, who make the local decisions in planning and development following the central decisions by the Ministry of Health and Social Welfare.

During the same period of time, ambulatory PHC was made free of charge and is now financed by taxation. Approximately half of the costs are covered by state tax revenue. The average total cost per inhabitant for primary health care was estimated to be USD600.

Specialised care in Finland is provided and financed in the same manner by communes, the country being divided into 21 districts for specialised care. The planning systems and administration structures for PHC and specialised care are different, thus primary health care is independent of specialised care.

The centralised planning system of the Ministry of Health and Social

Welfare, is based on a 5 year planning cycle which is revised annually; a process that made it possible to increase resources for PHC substantially compared to the increase in resources for specialised care. The upper limit in the increase of resources has been defined centrally for each district. During the period of 1972-1987, there was an increase from 17,000 to 50,000 health care workers within PHC, whereas the increase during the same period of time within the specialised care was only of 7000. This increase in the volume of PHC resulted in construction of health centres in the communes. These health centres were planned and built by people often more familiar with the hospital world than the needs of PHC. This resulted in the health centres being built and organised as small hospitals, working more or less on an 'assembly-line' basis, instead of an institution trying to see the patient as a whole.

In 1981, the Ministry of Health and Social Welfare began to plan in a more effective way to organise PHC services. Projects were undertaken to evaluate effects of different kinds of organisational models based on experiences in United Kingdom, Netherlands and Denmark. The first projects conducted between 1985-1987, have shown marked improvement in the provision of primary medical care services. A decentralised responsibility with a clearly defined framework for operating with a clearly defined population has been shown to improve continuity of care and patient and staff satisfaction. These projects concentrated on primary medical care only. Whereby the responsibility for the provision of care was transferred from the health centre to physicians who became responsible personally for a defined population; the personal doctor scheme.

The next step in Finland is to combine the personal doctor idea with other types of services - that is by turning primary care into primary health care. A set of new projects have begun 1990 to evaluate different approaches, which are expected to be completed by 1995. By then it should be possible to see whether or not these new and different approaches have transformed primary health care in Finland.

The report which follows documents the attempt in one health district to move towards a more integrated form of primary health care.

Managing decentralization of primary health care

Pertti Soveri and Asta Stenvall

Primary Health Care services for the health centre District of Porvoo have been sub-divided into 8 smaller sections, serving populations of 3500-7000. The purpose of this sub-division was to see if decentralisation of PHC services to small semi-autonomous units would result in a better quality service for patients. The effect of these administrative changes on the coverage of services, continuity of care, accessibility and utilisation of services, health, behaviour and satisfaction of the population and satisfaction of the health care workers is discussed.

Background

The public health centre of Porvoo provides PHC services for the population of 4 communes, Askola, Pornainen, the city of Porvoo and the rural commune of Porvoo. The population (1990) by commune is respectively: 4180; 3049; 20,296; and 20,271. Slightly over half (51.5%) of the population are women. About 13% of the population is aged 65 and over and this proportion is projected to rise to 15.5% by 2010.

Approximately 42,000 of the population live within the area of the main health centre, where the hospital beds, laboratory and x-ray services, rehabilitation and the on-call services are situated. The remaining 7000 inhabitants live in two small communes which, at the beginning of the project, were operating on a geographically defined population responsibility basis for PHC services. In these communes, the health staff were responsible for providing the necessary PHC services for the inhabitants, whereas in the main health centre staff were responsible collectively for providing these services for all the 42000 population.

The economical structure of the district consists of agriculture and foresting (4.2%), industries and construction (43.3%) and service sector (52.5%). The unemployment rate has varied between 2.5%-3.5% during the last few years.

A noted geographical feature of Porvoo District is the long shore line and the archipelago, which presents some difficulties in providing services in wintertime depending on ice formation and weather conditions. The population consists almost totally of Finnish citizens. No other ethnic groups of minorities are represented except for some Vietnamese families that have been placed within the district during the last three years.

The health centre employs approximately 400 employees, of which 35 are physicians. In the beginning of the project, four of the physicians worked outside the main health centre in the two small communes Askola and Pornainen.

Aims of the project

A problem with a large centralised unit is the lack of personal involvement in patient care. Patients see too many different physicians for too many different reasons, resulting in overlapping examinations, medications and unnecessary contacts with poor continuity of care. This leads to poor motivation for work and diminished responsibility for the care of the patient. Dissatisfaction between workers and patients increases leading to the feeling among some patients of being no more than an object on an 'assembly-line'. Furthermore, intersectoral cooperation and cooperation between health care and medical care is also poor.

A centralised unit situated on one particular place is not very efficient in taking care of socio-medical problems. Geographic separation leads to lack of knowledge about the social structures of families, problems within different housing areas, schools and other factors influencing health within an area, for instance traffic and construction.

The potential to react to the health problems of specific areas or population groups is impeded where there is no clear responsibility to take care of such populations. Neither is there enough knowledge based on evaluation or research of the health problems of smaller areas.

Research shows that smaller health services delivery where there is a clear framework of responsibility and team work, improves health care worker satisfaction and continuity of care for patients (Gray, 1979; Vohlonen, 1989; Evans & McBride, 1968). The purpose of this project was to see if decentralisation of all ambulatory PHC services to smaller independent units would bring beneficial effects to both patients and health workers.

Decentralisation in Porvoo

The city of Porvoo and the rural commune of Porvoo was gradually divided into six small districts during the years 1986-1989. The size of the new districts were determined by the need of personnel resources and availability of personnel in relation to the population size of the District. A balance was sought between a unit not being too small to be vulnerable in cases of absences due to illness and the population not being too big to prevent working in close contact with individual patients in productive team work.

The general assumption has been that depending upon the nature of the tasks, a physician can take care of a population of 1200-2500 inhabitants. If providing only medical services, a physician generally can take care of a population of 1800-2500. However, adding obligations like preventive health care, and provision of services schools reduces the physician patient ratio towards the lower end of the range. In Porvoo all physicians took part in all PHC activities, resulting in a population of 1200-1400 per physician.

For a unit to be able to function adequately there should be at least two physicians present at all times. Physicians in Finland are away from their duties approximately 30% of the year due to vacations, studies and leaves of absence. This means that normally, without locums, one of three physicians is always absent. Taking into account the unexpected absences and periods of postgraduate studies, there must be at least four physicians in a unit to ensure that two of them are always present if the unit is to operate without locums. Accordingly it was decided to have four to five physicians in every unit. This meant that the unit population size would be approximately 6000-7000. Each unit also should have approximately two nurses, two district nurses, three health visitors and four auxiliary staff, although exact numbers vary according to the social and age structure of the area.

These units would have responsibility and authority to provide all primary medical care services except for out of hours on call service for their population. Additionally they provide health care services during pregnancy, for children and schools, day care centres and elderly people. Nursing homes and home care for elderly and chronically ill patients are part of the work, as is taking samples for laboratory analyses. Each unit has its own budget and has freedom to operate within the framework of the budget and the working plan approved by the political board controlling the parent health centre.

Methods for evaluation

The effect of these administrative changes was evaluated according to several parameters:

* Continuity of care was measured with an index calculated from the computerised patient records by the following procedure:
  number of visits - number of physicians + 1 divided by the

number of visits. This gives an index from 0 to 1, where 1 represents the ideal; that all visits are made by the same doctor.

* Coverage of the services was calculated by dividing the number of users by the number of inhabitants.

* Accessibility was measured by comparing changes in waiting times for appointments and changes in consumption of services.

* Client health, behaviour and satisfaction was measured annually each September by an anonymous questionnaire. The first was administered in September 1988. The sample population was standardised for age and gender. The sample size was 600 in 1988 and 1000 in 1989 and 1990. In the future the client satisfaction questionnaire will take place at three yearly intervals.

* Health care worker satisfaction was measured every three years with a questionnaire. The questionnaire, with 33 different questions, measures the changes in the 'atmosphere' of the working environment on a scale of 1 to 10.

Results

Continuity of care, expressed as the percentage of clients where the continuity index was more than 0.5, increased markedly during the 2 first years and then has remained relatively stable. The percentages for 1985 and 1986 were calculated from samples of 200 randomly chosen clients, whereas the percentages for the following years were calculated from the computerised patient records and include all patients that visited the health centre. Patients with only one visit were excluded. The yearly trend was as follows:

1985	25.8%
1986	30.8%
1987	37.9%
1988	38.0%
1989	35.3%

Continuity of care was better in the units situated away from the main health centre, where 41%-66% of the patients had an index of more than

0.5, compared with the mean (approximately 0.38) for the whole health centre.

Coverage of services remained largely the same during the period of the project. Any differences that occurred were affected by the available number of physicians working hours. The number of visits made outside regular working hours as compared to the total number of visits did not change. This was partly due to limited capacity available during regular working hours. The lack of locums in 1989 showed markedly in the consumption statistics.

Accessibility as measured in waiting time for an appointment varied between 9 and 11 days. No marked changes were observed as a result of the decentralised experiment.

The questionnaire measuring patient health, behaviour and satisfaction showed no major changes during the evaluation period. Responses varied between 73%-77%. One reminder only was sent to the sample population. About one third of the respondents had a personal doctor which, in slightly more than half of the cases, was at the health centre. Just over half of the people visited the health centre in case of acute illness, instead of other surgeries. No major change in perceived levels of health was observed. The percentage of those who estimated that health care services within the district had not changed or had improved, remained constant.

Health care worker satisfaction increased slightly during the evaluation period. On a scale from 1 to 10, the increase during the observation period rose from 5.3 to 6.0 for the whole health centre and to 6.5 for the unit that had been set up away from the main health centre.

Discussion

Decentralisation of PHC can be affected in several different ways. The method chosen in Porvoo was based on a geographic format and population size in which a small team with a clearly defined framework of responsibility and authority administers the PHC services. In this context, the team provides all PHC services for its population, without the assistance of the main health centre. This approach differs somewhat from the personal doctor projects administered by the Ministry of Health and Social Welfare (Ministry of Health and Social Welfare, 1986; Helenius, 1987; Levike, 1989), in which the responsibility for a patients health is put on a more individual level. Some of the projects use geographical frameworks, some a more flexible approach whereby the patient can more freely choose his/her physician in a way similar to that in the United Kingdom and Denmark.

The main difference between the Porvoo model and the personal doctors projects is that patient work in Porvoo is based on team work, where different types of needs are tackled by different members of the team according to their experience and professional backgrounds.

The decentralisation is not total. A certain amount of guidance and control is administered by the health centre to maintain equity in the provision of services between the different units. Theses guidelines give financial and functional legitimacy to the daily activities. They are prepared by the units and approved by the health centre administration.

The operation of a unit and the outcome of its work must be monitored and evaluated. The unit expects certain results for its population and therefore must have information on the outcome of its plans and policies. Different parameters are evaluated in order to be able to follow and assess the effect of these administrative changes in Porvoo.

During the years 1985-1987 there was a marked improvement in continuity of care, together with greater health care personnel satisfaction, which suggests an improved quality of care. It was during these years that the main functional change from one health centre into smaller units took place. The observation times so far have been too short to show other significant changes especially as the administrative changes were not completed until the beginning of 1989. Only one new unit operated alongside the main health centre with two more units set up during 1991, at the end of the study period. This means that a much longer follow-up is necessary in order to detect changes in patient health, behaviour and satisfaction. However, it is possible to draw some conclusions as changes in patient satisfaction are not dependent entirely on organisational changes.

This is because the questionnaire used in the Porvoo study partly measures the same parameters as the country wide study (Kalivo, *et al*, 1989), which gives an opportunity to make comparisons with other areas in Finland. The findings for Porvoo in patient health, behavioural and satisfaction are consistent with the findings of the country wide study.

The main problem which has inhibited the administrative changes from achieving their effect has been the difficult locum situation for physicians. In 1989, there was a 20% decrease in available physician time. This meant increased stress for the organisation and a resulting handicap in providing the needed services.

The evaluation methodology appears sufficient for the needs of the health centre. The sampling interval however seems to be too short. The results presented here are mainly for the health centre. The same factors are being analyzed at unit level and will be presented later. Overall, these observations suggest an improvement in health care services and correlate with the increased quality of care observed elsewhere (Ministry of Health and Social Welfare, 1986; Vohlonen, 1989; Kekki, 1982; Evans, 1968).

Ireland

Primary health care

The Republic of Ireland has a population of approximately 3.5 million. The population has an unusually young age structure, with 30.3% in the 0-14 year age group and only 10.7% over 65s. Since 1980 the birth rate has been falling, and the total period fertility rate is now approximately 2.1. The relative and absolute number of elderly will grow in the coming decades. Life expectancy is at the lower end of European norms: in 1980-1982, at birth a male could expect to live to 70.1 years and a female to 75.6 years; at age 65 a male could expect to live a further 12.6 years and a female 15.7 years.

Ireland has a low population density and little heavy industry. Many of the environmental problems in mainland Europe are less acute here. Lifestyle factors show large areas where health could be improved: 32% of over 15s smoke; alcohol consumption has been rising, although per capita consumption is not high on European standards; diet is out of line with recommended intakes, particularly for total and saturated fat intake. Immunisation against measles, mumps, rubella, pertussis, diphtheria, tetanus and polio is provided and uptakes are improving, although reliable national figures for absolute levels are not available.

There are marked socio-economic gradients in morbidity and mortality. There is, however, no consistent geographical pattern. Premature deaths, particularly from cardiovascular disease lower the life expectancy; between 1965 and 1984, admissions to psychiatric hospitals for alcoholism increased by 339%. Deaths in road traffic accidents have fallen marginally in recent years. Infant mortality has fallen to under 9 per 1000.

The present structure for the health services was set up by the 1970 Health Act. Public expenditure on health grew rapidly in the 1970s and reached nearly 7.5% of GNP in the early 1980s. Since then expenditure has been sharply reduced both in real terms and as a percent of GNP. During this period, community services were supposed to be protected and a policy of shifting the emphasis to PHC adopted, although this did not always occur. The primary medical services, which were operating on an open ended fee per item system increased rapidly in cost and therefore consumed a greater proportion of PHC resources. Under the Programme for Economic and Social Progress, the government has promised real increases in expenditure on PHC services over the next seven years.

There are eight health boards in the Republic of Ireland through which health and welfare services are delivered. Each Health Board covers a number of local authority areas and vary in population from 1.2 million to 202,000. The governing boards are composed of a mixture of local authority representatives, nominees of the Minister of Health, and representatives of the health professions, most of whom are medical practitioners. The elected local representatives form a majority on the board.

The boards' services are usually delivered through three programmes: community care programme, special hospital programme; and, general hospital programme. The boards co-operate with a wide range of voluntary bodies some of which they grant aid. Services in the community are delivered through community care areas with populations of approximately 100,000 each. In each community care area there is a community care team. The primary medical service is delivered through general practitioners who are independent contractors with the health boards and they usually do not work in partnerships. They are paid under a mainly capitation based system which was only introduced in March 1989. Those entitled to this service (medical card holders) receive this service (and any drugs prescribed) free of charge. Nursing and paramedical staff are normally attached to the health board rather than to individual general practitioners. Services in the special hospital programme have been undergoing a rapid transformation in recent years in accordance with a policy of moving patients from institutional to community settings.

Hospitals delivering secondary and tertiary care services are usually run by the health boards in country areas. In the larger urban centres however, many hospitals are run by hospital boards independent of the health boards. These may be 'voluntary' (usually run by religious orders) or statutory boards appointed directly by the Minister of Health. They receive their funding directly from the Department of Health.

Eligibility for public health services in Ireland has recently been simplified. It was agreed to extend eligibility for free hospital consultant services to everyone. Approximately a third of the population take out a policy for private sickness insurance with the Voluntary Health Insurance Board which is a semi-state body providing insurance on a community rating principle. This covers private treatment both in private hospitals and in private wards in public hospitals.

The allocation of resources has largely been based on a historical cost plus basis with some new services being specifically funded. The Irish health services have always trained more health professionals than are required, and consequently Ireland continues to export trained health personnel. Associated with this training, much research is conducted. There is a national Health Research Board, but this is poorly funded and the majority of research funding comes from other sources. Development of information systems in the health service is progressing, but a considerable investment is still required.

An organisational and managerial model for the decentralised delivery of services

Chris Buttanshaw and Fred Donahue

The overall aim of the proposed changes to the Eastern Health Board is to establish the optimum organisational and managerial model for the decentralisation delivery of services. Implicit in this is the belief that the delivery of efficient, equitable and effective health care requires such a system.

Background

The Eastern Health Board (EHB) area comprises the three counties of Dublin, Kildare and Wicklow, and with a population of 1.232 million is by far the largest health board in the Republic. The population has a young age distribution, with 30% in the age range 0-14. Only 8.7% of the population were aged over 65 in 1986. Between 1981 and 2006 it has been estimated that Board's population aged over 65s will rise by 33%, and the number over 75 by 43%. The relatively greater health service resource consumption seen in these age groups means that careful planning will be required to meet the anticipated extra demands. The balance between PHC services and other services is central to this process.

The search for a new structure

The need for a reorganisation of the delivery of health care in Ireland has been widely recognised. In 1987, the Minister of Health set up a Commission to examine the funding of health services, and a national working party to examine the future role of community medicine. Their reports recognised the need for better systems for evaluating services and measuring health needs and outcomes. At the same time the Board was critically examining its own structures. The problems identified were as follows:

*   The lack of integration between the various EHB programmes, the general practitioner service and the rest of the Board's health services; and between the Board's services and those of other sectoral and voluntary bodies, particularly voluntary hospitals;

*   The centralisation of many functions and decision making processes;
*   The lack of objective measures of health need;
*   The lack of measures of outcome of health service activities;
*   Inadequate involvement of the recipients of services in the structure.

An outline proposal for the reorganisation of the EHB has been approved in principal. The approach has been to plan a new locality structure for the board, and then to work towards the more central district structure, rather than the more usual process which works in the opposite direction. The key concepts behind the proposal for such a new structure are equity, decentralisation, community participation, integration of services with an emphasis on PHC, and information systems containing measures of need and measures of outcome.

The essential step in this reorganisation was the creation of a locally based system that would be responsive to people's needs in the community. From consideration of the situation in the Board's area, a review of the international situation and comparison with the experience of TTB colleagues, localities of 25,000 population approximately seem to be optimum; being neither too large to lose the benefits of decentralisation and local identity, nor so small that administration of services at that level would be impractical. The smallest unit of population in Ireland is the District Electoral Division (DED). Thus, the localities have been formed by grouping DEDs. Each locality so formed can also be seen as a number of neighbourhoods, and below the locality level service delivery can be tailored to these neighbourhoods. The principles followed in drawing locality boundaries were as follows:

*   Boundaries must follow DED lines;
*   Neighbourhoods with a sense of identity should not be divided;
*   Natural boundaries should be followed as far as possible;
*   Locality populations should fall in the 25,000 to 30,000 range, unless there was an atypical need profile, or marked demographic change was expected;
*   Localities are drawn with existing transport networks in mind;
*   Localities must be capable of being grouped into general hospital catchments based on the most convenient hospital;
*   Localities should not straddle local authority boundaries.

Following these principles, the Board's area has been divided up into 45 localities. Each locality has a headquarters which is a 'one stop shop' for all the Board's services. In addition, where possible, other sectoral public bodies, and voluntary organisations would be based in the same premises.

In each locality there is a public health team, which would have a side ranging remit in health promotion, the monitoring of need, planning of services to meet that need, delivery of certain community services, and the measurement of health outcomes for their locality population. The locality is responsible for monitoring both its own services and also services provided to its population by other units or agencies. In time budgetary structures will be devised to include use of hospital or specialised service. The measurement of need for and outcome of hospital services will be a function of the locality.

Within the overall district and Board policies, the locality is responsible for its health promotion work. Each locality is expected, in particular, to develop close working relationships with local community in the decisions making process. The staffing of each district will be determined by an agreed need formula. The factors considered wold include the age and sex structure of the population, socio-economic variable and mortality indicators. One particularly important area is the integration of general practitioners (GPs) with the bulk of their PHC colleagues. The formal linking of GPs into the locality structure is not possible because of their independent contractor status in the health system, and the large proportion of private practice. GP's practices are not geographically defined and will continue to span across the locality boundaries. However, the locality headquarters is positioned so that it is easily accessible for all of that locality population, making it an ideal location for GP's as well.

Districts

While the function of the Board is delegated to the locality as far as possible, the locality could not function as a stand alone unit. The 45 localities thus formed are gathered into districts to form six district management units. Each of these districts contains a general hospital, or complex of general hospitals. Within each district there is a district care team composed of the heads of the various disciplines as well as hospital representation. The hospitals, in time, will become units serving the localities and they would then be held accountable to the locality manager for their performance in meeting agreed obligations. The hospital budget would then be determined by the population needs it is contracted to meet.

Research undertaken by Corcoran and O'Shea (1989) has examined two groups of elderly persons deemed to be on the margin of domiciliary and institutional care. Significant factors of importance in determining the current placement of these elderly people were identified. The formal and informal costs of institutional and community care were estimated and conclusions drawn; namely, that the treatment of informal care as a free good was inappropriate.

The localities at the centre of the Board's services for the elderly. They plan and co-ordinate all services for the elderly in their catchment and deliver PHC services through their multidisciplinary teams. The piloting of these structures for the care of the elderly was planned for the new South West district, but because of the priority that services for the aged have come to assume, new resources have been made available to develop community services for them.

During a transitional period, these services are being delivered through the existing Community Care Areas (CCAs). Each of the ten CCAs are setting up a 'Community Ward' scheme, and in the five CCAs with the greatest elderly populations, two such Wards are being formed. These community wards 'admit' elderly patients in need of community health services, and provide an enhanced and expanded range of services designed to maximise health and opportunities for continuing community care.

The populations of the catchment areas for these wards will, in time, come to be coterminous with the localities, but initially will be larger. Each CCA will have a multidisciplinary team representative of the community care services, the psychiatric services, the general hospital services, and the housing services. This body will be responsible for the overall co-ordination and planning services for the aged. These functions eventually will be subsumed under the district care team in the new proposals.

Under these teams there are locality teams for the elderly, initially dedicated to services for elderly patients who have been admitted to the 'community ward'. These are multidisciplinary; including physiotherapists, occupational therapists, public health nurses, state registered nurses, nurses aides and home helps, and headed up by a public health nurse who would usually have senior status. Thus these new teams will pilot some aspects of the locality system, and the team dynamics that are required.

Epidemiological information system

In order to devise the new structures, information concerning the health, demography and welfare of the population was required at a local level. The Board has been working on a system to produce such information, the Epidemiological Information System (EIS). In time, it is intended that all significant information relating to the health of populations in small areas will be included.

One widely used measure for determining resource allocation has been the standardised mortality ratio (SMR). The EIS has been used to plot for 1986-1989 mortality in the Dublin area. The results have been used to identify areas with a higher than expected mortality (Johnson *et al* 1989). A research group was set up to investigate the relationship between the SMR and conventional risk factors for premature mortality. Some 354 adults aged 25-44 from areas with high mortality were compared with 333 from low mortality areas. In high mortality ares 51% were current smokers compared to 29% in low mortality areas. Adults in these areas were also more likely to take inadequate exercise and eat an unhealthy diet (Johnson *et al* 1991). This work has validated the use of SMRs as a proxy measure for need for health activities in small areas.

Births in the Dublin area are being coded to DEDs along with certain perinatal information, A profile of the number of births, the perinatal mortality and the average birth weight for DEDs has been devised. This information is being obtained from the Central Statistics Office, and will be available to plan resource allocation, particularly for child care services. In time, the information will become directly available to the EHB from its implementation of the RICHs software which will register all births along with perinatal information, and include information on immunisation and use of other child health services.

As an initial measure of morbidity, it is intended to include data on drug prescribing from the medical card scheme. Initial analysis is available for some of the data on drug prescribing. An index of quality of prescribing on PHC is being devised and this will be an important quality indicator for primary health care.

Public health nursing

This new structure envisages the expansion of the role of the Public Health Nurse (PHN). A study was undertaken to document the activities of PHNs in a Community Care Area and to evaluate their role. The situation regarding community nursing nationally and internationally was reviewed. Instruments were devised to document PHN activity and to evaluate the attitudes of GPs, hospital consultants, and hospital ward sisters. Unfortunately, the PHNs declined to return the instrument, and thus, so far, this important part of the study has not been evaluated.

Some 88.6% of GPs were satisfied with the quality of care in the PHN service, but satisfaction was less in regard to communication, access to service and out of hours service, Similarly ward sisters and consultants were dissatisfied with the out of hours service. The referral behaviour to PHNs for a variety of services/therapies was ascertained and the preference in each case between a PHN, a State Registered Nurse (SRN - a nurse without specialist community nursing qualifications), and a nurses aide. In all cases, there was felt to be room for certain services/therapies to be carried out by SRNs or nurses aides. The study conclusions were:

*   SRNs and nurses aides should be introduced into community nursing;

*   There should be regular formal and informal contact between the PHN and the GP;

*   A liaison PHN should develop links with all hospitals (at present liaison nurses have been appointed for some hospitals only);

*   A twilight nursing service (out of hours nursing) should be introduced.

Community participation

Community participation is crucial to the success of the locality model. Different structures are being tried in different localities in the South West District and the experience of the other TTB participants was particularly helpful in this regard. In addition, valuable lessons have been gained in this area from the following three projects:

Ballymun project: Ballymun is a deprived area to the North of Dublin. There have been ongoing problems associated with social deprivation, high unemployment and a rapid turnover of local authority tenants. The Ballymun Community Coalition, which is an umbrella organisation for the many voluntary and community groups, has been formed. This coalition has catalysed the formation of a task force consisting of the Coalition, the Local Authority, the EHB and national elected representatives. This task force has reported on the problems facing Ballymun and made wide ranging recommendations on possible solutions, including a multi-million pound refurbishment of the flat complexes and the surrounding lands. Its proposal, in a phased form, has been approved by the national Department of the Environment and work has begun on the first phase.

Blanchardstown project: Three large new satellite towns have been developed to the West of Dublin. These share many problems related to poor infrastructure and lack of social cohesion. The development of successful PHC depends upon, and influences, the social structure of the community. To address this, the EHB has participated in a community development project in one of these towns, the Greater Blanchardstown Project. This project has developed programmes promoting personal and community development. Evaluation of these programmes showed that participants self-esteem increased and that they were more likely to participate in community activities. Thus the model has been shown to be a successful method of improving community health.

Community mothers scheme: The Community Mothers Scheme demonstrates the mechanisms whereby the community itself can provide services and participate directly in improving its own health, in this case by improving parenting skills and capabilities. Specially trained PHNs recruited mothers in disadvantaged communities and provided them with skills to visit and assist other mothers in their own neighbourhood. This project has grown from limited experimental beginnings, to cover all Community Care Areas and involve over 1000 sets of (mostly first time) parents (there are c.19,000 births in the Board's area). The project is a valuable demonstration of one model for health promotion initiatives in the localities.

Portugal

Primary health care

Portugal has had PHC services since 1971 through the public health centres network. PHC services are available to 100% of the population, and more than 50% use the services. In 1989, there were 343 public PHC centres managed by 18 Regional Health Administrations, acting for the PHC Central Department. PHC depends heavily on the private sector. In 1986, 38% of PHC total expenditure was spent on direct provision of services (preventive and curative activities), while the remaining 62% were transferred to the private sector.

The main providers of PHC are GPs (1/1622 inhabitants) and public health doctors and nurses. However, there are significant differences in the geographical distribution of health professionals. In the services it provides, PHC is mainly engaged in disease prevention and cure, and referring patients to other levels of care. There is no community participation at PHC level. Several intersectoral co-operation programmes have been developed at the central level, concerning nutrition, traffic accidents, smoking and cardiovascular diseases.

Since 1970, the population has grown at a rate of about 18%, due to immigration and people returning from the former colonies. The population is relatively young in comparison with other European countries. In 1987, 12.5% of the population were over 65 years old. Life expectancy at birth was 70 years for men, and 76.9 years for women.

In 1985, environmental sanitation provided safe water for 60% of population and water sanitation systems for 40%. According to national health statistics, the Portuguese diet contains too much protein and fat, mainly animal fat, and too little carbohydrates and fibre, as compared with a recommended diet. In 1988, 33% of the population smoked (men 50%; women 14%). There has been a National Vaccination Programmed since the late 1960's.

Portugal has the highest mortality rates in the EU for infectious diseases; Cerebro-vascular diseases; motor vehicle accidents; and stomach cancer; and the second highest for liver cirrhosis.

Infant mortality rate (1988) was 13.0/1000 live births. A morbidity study in 1987, indicated that over a two week period, about 6% of the population was sick in bed, and about one in four persons were potential users of the health services.

Between 1975 and 1987, total expenditure for health, as a percentage of gross domestic product remained at roughly the same level of 6.4 percent the public proportion being 3.8% in 1975 and 3.9% in 1987. In 1988, investment on PHC services represented 13.9% of total expenditure on health services, while that on secondary care represented 82.5%

Indicators to improve decision-making and resource allocation process

Walter Adrahi, Carlos Costa Neves and Luis Brito de Azevedo.

Following the strategy to influence the local planning and decision-making processes to achieve efficient use of resources available, this project aims at improving the decision making process in PHC by providing local health authorities with efficient instruments for collecting and analysing health data. Specifically, it is expected that the project will provide more and better information for local planning and monitoring, as well as for regional budgeting; and more control and choice over use of local resources to meet local needs.

In 1989, it was decided to select seven health indicators, using the Delphi and Nominal Group techniques, to provide local health authorities with information for planning and decision making. Five health centres monitored and evaluated these indicators. The evaluation was completed at the beginning of 1991. Some of the first selected indicators were shown to be not appropriate to creating changes in local health management. However, a new dynamic was introduced in the daily life of the health centres involved, in that staff were encouraged to periodically evaluate their work. As a result, the Regional Department of Health decided to introduce periodic review using a revised list of selected indicators.

Background

The Azores in an archipelago of nine islands with a resident population of 240,000. The Azorean health care system consists of fifteen health centres, one for each administrative council, and three hospitals located in the main islands. Every health service has its own administration, and operational regulations. Each hospital is economically and administratively autonomous, with resources allocated directly from the Regional Government and not influenced by a needs-based formula. Health care in the Azores is free. Hospital care is secondary and complementary to primary health care.

The health system faces several challenges: increasing health care costs; health administration needs to be strengthened to meet increasing health demands; the pace and costs of technological development, indispensable to the improvement of the quality of care, exceeds the financial capacities of the Azorean government; resource rationalisation and allocation cannot follow the same methods that could be adopted in the mainland, due to the insularity of the Region.

Health services are changing in order to reduce social and geographical inequalities and improve the quality and efficiency of the services. Decentralisation is being adopted as a management strategy to improve efficiency. The curative and hospital centred system is being replaced by the PHC based system. The main aims are: first, to extend the number of health centres in which multi-disciplinary teams (doctors, nurses and social workers), provide preventive and curative care, with sufficient administrative and technical support, to well defined populations; and second, to implement of the family doctor system and PHC lists. The process involves the establishment of specific units for management of PHC at local and regional levels, responsible both for PHC services and health promotion activities.

Traditionally, health services planning has followed an incrementalist model, without explicit objectives, using normative rigid decision-making processes. This, added to unequal accessibility of population groups to decision levels, resulted in an imbalance of services not sufficiently responsive to needs. Regionalisation, setting of targets, capital investment plans and programme budgeting are tools that are slowly beginning to change the system.

The resource allocation process has been based solely on indicators of utilisation of health services. Now that the installation of PHC services is almost completed, equity principles of resource allocation should be adopted. The following criteria are important for the equitable delivery of health services: the health needs of the population; coverage by health services; assurance of minimum health care activities.

Some data has been available through different systems without correlation or links to PHC services. Utilization and morbidity data are of low quality and generally not useful for health planning and evaluation. Mortality and resources information are not available, and thus the creation of appropriate systems is required.

Methodology

Delphi and Nominal group techniques were used to identify useful health indicators for local health planning and decision making. Five Delphi Panels and one Nominal Group meeting were carried out by mail, and were made up of a minimum of 20 health professionals (physicians, nurses and administrators) from five health centres where selected indicators could be measures and tested. The last Delphi Panel, was carried out in a meeting of all fifteen managers of health centres. The

Nominal Group was formed by a group of persons strategically placed in the Health Department and other health-related sectors (namely, health and social services professionals, regional politicians, community and religious leaders, and journalists).

The first Panel determined which indicators health professionals thought were most useful for planning and decision-making at local level; whether those indicators were already available or not; and if not available, how they thought they could be made available. At the second stage, the staff of the five health centres collected data concerning the chosen indicators, using either special surveys or the regional-based health statistic system. The following sources were used to obtain the data: vital events registers; population and housing censuses; routine health services records; epidemiological surveillance data; sample surveys; disease registers; and data from sectors other than health. The second, third and fourth Panels aimed at reducing the initial list of 31 indicators to seven, based on information about successes and problems in data collection and analysis.

The Nominal Group also aimed at identifying its own list of seven health indicators useful for planning and decision making in PHC. In a meeting facilitated by a health professional, the members of the Nominal Group were asked to list the 20 most important regional health problems. In successive rounds, after information and discussion about problems in data collection and analysis, the members were asked to reduce and specify the initial list.

More than one year after the first Panel, a fifth Panel was carried out, to evaluate the initial list of indicators and both methods of getting information for better decisions in PHC (routine statistics and special surveys). This Panel also compared the results of the previous stages and the results of the Nominal Group meeting.

Results

The indicators selected by the Delphi Panels and the Nominal Group are presented in Table 7. The seven indicators selected by the fourth Panel are marked D4; the seven indicators selected by the Nominal Group are marked NG; the indicators selected by the fifth Panel, after evaluation of the initial indicators, are marked D5.

The indicators selected initially were related to the World Health Organization Regional Targets. Following the selection process, regional and local health authorities and the health centre managers involved in this study tried, for two years, to monitor the chosen indicators (D4). The results of monitoring the indicators revealed that these had limited impact on the management of health centres. It was necessary to select better indicators to assist in the development of health services in the Azores. To achieve this, the fifth Delphi Panel was established in 1991, and selected the indicators (D5) to be monitored in the next two years.

In a period of changing profiles of morbidity and morality, it was recognised that indicators monitoring local health services are important. However, the choice of indicators has not been easy and the fist seven health indicators were not readily accepted. At the outset, there had been a tendency to choose health impact indicators rather than those related to health impact and efficiency. In the initial list, the majority of the indicators are future oriented rather than present oriented and try to ascertain progress according to PHC principles of community participation, health education, integration of preventive activities, teamwork and increased PHC weight in the overall health services. In the final list, it can be seen that there is a clear tendency to emphasize the factors that may contribute to the improvement of the day-to-day management of health centres.

However, information on changing patterns of health is now better understood and improvement in the collection of data through death certificates and other systems now begins to provide the necessary information for the development of indicators to improve monitoring resource allocation. The project has increased the interest in monitoring and selecting indicators. The impact of this work is seen in the stimulus and motivation of participants, especially local stimulus and motivation of participants, especially local workers. The researchers beleive that the use of methodology that allows local people to participate in the design of the information system is essential for the process to be successful.

Table 7
Indicators selected by delphi panels and nominal group

Indicator	d1	d2	d3	d4	ng	d5
1 General mortality rate	*	*	*	*	*	*
2 Disease-specific mortality rate	*	*				
3 Proportionate mortality from specific diseases	*	*	*	*	*	*
4 Infant mortality rate	*	*				
5 Perinatal mortality rate	*					*
6 Maternal mortality rate	*	*	*	*		
7 Child mortality rate	*					
8 Morbidity	*	*				*
9 Disability	*	*	*	*		*
10 Percentage of immunised children < 7 years old	*	*	*	*	*	*
11 Immunisation rate for rubella < 14 years old	*					
12 Percentage of population > 65 years old receiving health care	*	*	*	*	*	*
13 Percentage of population lying in bed receiving domiciliary health care	*					*
14 Percentage of pregnants receiving health care	*	*	*	*	*	
15 Percentage of primary school children attended by PHC team	*	*				*
16 Percentage of school children transferred to hospitals	*					*

Continued ...

.... Table 7 continued

Indicator	d1	d2	d3	d4	ng	d5
17 Percentage of population 14-17 years old receiving health care in PHC lists)	*	*	*			*
18 Average waiting time for a consultation	*	*				*
19 Average waiting time for a consultation in the waiting room	*	*				
20 Transference of patients to another island/mainland	*	*				*
21 Absenteeism in days per health centre and per year	*	*	*		*	
22 Percentage of pensioners among 16-64 year olds	*	*	*		*	*
23 Average cost of a consultation	*	*				*
24 Average cost of a PHC team domiciliary visit	*					
25 Average cost of PHC nurse domiciliary visit	*					
26 Average cost of chronic patient day in the health centre (+90 days)	*					*
27 Average cost of other patient day in the health centre	*					
28 Bed occupation by chronic patients in the health centre	*	*				*
29 Average bed occupation in the patients internment	*					
30 Percentage of false emergencies	*					
31 No of prescriptions per consultation	*	*	*			

d1 = 1st delphi panel, d2 = 2nd, d3 = 3rd, d4 = 4th, d5 = 5th,
ng = nominal group

Evaluation of the quality of medical referral to a mental health clinic

Delfim Cardoso and Fidalgo Freitas

An innovation in intra-sectoral collaboration in relation to Mental Health is described. This project recognised that the quality of mental health referral was poor and so special training was provided for general practitioners to improve the quantity and quality of their work on mental health. A protocol of good practice was developed and, on later evaluation of its use, it was found that both quantity and quality of referral by GP's to Specialists was improving.

The objectives of the study were fourfold: to evaluate the quantity and quality of medical referral between GP's and the Centre of Mental Health, and its evolution in time; to evaluate the evolution of pathology in the population and its geographical distribution; to evaluate changes in first referral of patients; and, to suggest a course of action according to the results of these evaluations.

Background

Viseu is a mountainous district in North Eastern Portugal with a population of 427,400 inhabitants. The District is divided into twenty four counties, some of which are more than 90 km from the District capital. About 50% of the population works in the Agricultural Sector (compared to the national average of 18%). In 1986, 44.2% of the population had water supplies, and only 25% were served by sewers. The main causes of death are cardio-vascular diseases. Alcoholism is also a major problem, affecting about 6% of the population. The District has three General Hospitals (Viseu, Lamego, and Tondela), seventy four PHC units, a hospital for Service of Pulmonary Diseases and a Centre of Mental Health (C.M.H.). In 1984, the CMH had forty acute beds, an ambulatory service in Viseu and Lamego, and a home support service for psychotic patients. It has two psychiatrists, twenty eight nurses and two social service technicians.

A number of major problems (scarcity of resources, which affected the functioning of the Centre; GP's not recognising symptoms of patients suffering from emotional distress; and the implementation of a new GPs career regulation) have led to the establishment of an information and development strategy that would improve the professional skills of medical professionals involved and facilitate the interchange between the two levels of care, PHC and Mental Health Care. Medical referral between GP's and the Mental Health Centre is an appropriate indicator of the quantitative and qualitative level of such interchange. Therefore, a protocol was developed and evaluated during 1987-1990 to stimulate and improve medical referral.

Methodology

The study was both longitudinal and retrospective. All clinical records of first visits to a psychiatrist, from 1984 to 1990, were reviewed according to the protocol: evaluations took place in 1987 and 1990. Data were collected from the psychiatric medical records. The variables in the research protocol included: general patient data (age, sex, marital situation, profession, area of residence); diagnosis; first referral; medical referral and quality; and patient destiny.

The definition of the concepts used in the study were the following:

*   First referral: Identification of the institution that first referred the patient to the Centre of Mental Health;

*   Medical referral: Clinical information that the patient brings with him to or from the Centre of Mental Health;

*   Content of medical referral:
                - Motive of the visit;
                - Description of symptoms;
                - Treatment and results;
                - Patient/family medical history;
                - Patient/family previous psychiatry history;
                - Previous diagnoses.

*   Type of medical referral:
                - Absent:When there is no medical referral;
                - Poor:When it includes only one of the items mentioned on content of the medical referral;
                - Regular:When it includes 2 of the items
                - Good:When it includes 3 or more of the items

Results

The study reviewed 1773 records of first visits to a psychiatrist, between 1984 and 1990; there was a maximum of 412 first visits in 1984, and a minimum of 94 visits in 1990. The majority of the patients were women (61%), and married (56%). About 68% of the cases were of patients aged between 21-60 years, and 20% of patients aged between 31-40 years. 42.8% of the patients came from the county of Viseu, the most populated and nearest to the Mental Health Centre. About 44% worked in Agriculture.

Depression was the most frequent diagnosis (56%), followed by schizophrenia (11%). The percentage of alcoholics in the clinic was low (4%), when contrasted with the District rank for this pathology - second in the country. The majority of the patients were referred to the CMH by their GP (31% on average), and this percentage has increased over the years from 12.7%, in 1984 to 47.9% in 1990. Over the same period, the percentage of those referred directly to the CMH, either by the family or by the local authority, has decreased.

There was a remarkable increase in the quantity and quality of medical referral over the years. In the latter years of the survey, 100% of patients referred to the CMH by GP's arrived with good quality medical referral. However, in looking at medical referral by diagnosis, in a large percentage of cases of psychosis manic-depressive relevant data was absent, and in cases of mental retardation it was of poor quality. In a high percentage of patients that were students, there was no indication of any professional status.

In the follow-up of the patients, after appropriate treatment, an average of 43.4% were referred back to the institution that sent them to the CMH. This percentage varied from 33.1% in 1984 to over 50% in 1990. There was also a significant decrease in patients abandoning treatment (24% on average), from 34.9% in 1984 to 9.5% in 1990.

Discussion and conclusion

Given the variables age, sex, marital status and psychiatry diagnosis, the results of this study were what could be expected in a psychiatric clinic. The percentage of patient that came from the agricultural sector (44%) is smaller than the percentage of the population working on this sector (50%). This may be explained in part by the fact that 42.8% of the patients came from the County of Viseu, the nearest, most populated and least rural county in the District.

A partial explanation for the low percentage of alcoholic patients that attend the CMH, may be that GP's generally take care of such cases. The Regional Centre for Alcoholism, in cooperation with the Regional Health Administration, has been conducting an intense activity of information and development of the GP's in this field.

The high percentage of missing medical referral details in the cases of psychoses manic-depressive may be because these patients often present to the services with an acute condition requiring treatment. The poor quality of medical referral in cases of mental retardation may be in part due to the patient's need for medical declarations and certificates for social purposes, rather than on clinical criteria.

The restructuring of the GPs career and the introduction of the technical and scientific development strategy, which stressed in all District the need for good quality medical referral as a means of achieving appropriate cooperation and coordination between services, may explain why the percentage of patients referred by GP's to the CMH was high (31%) and accounted for its steady increase over the years (from 12.7% to 47.9%). The high quantity and quality levels of medical referral also contributed to the creation of a climate of trust, resulting in a high number of patients (more than 50% in 1990), being referred back to the institution that sent them to CMH, and for the decline in the number that abandon treatment. This may also explain the decrease in the number of those attending the CMH by their own initiative, or through that of their family or the authorities.

There were a number of observations to come out of this project. First, there was a significant improvement on quantity and quality of medical referral in the period of the study, as well as improvement in the intersectoral cooperation between institutions. Second, the high levels of medical referral allowed for optimisation of provision of services, such as high accessibility and increased follow-up. Third, the strategy followed proved to be adequate to achieve the objectives of the activity. Fourth, in the context of intrasectoral cooperation and integration of PHC and Mental Health Care, this strategy seems not only relevant, but one that could be easily transferable to other districts.

Spain

Primary health care

Spain has a population of 40 million. After a steep rise in population growth in the 1960's it now has a growth of about 2.9% as a consequence of a continuously decreasing birth rate (10.84%, 1989) and a mortality rate of 7.97% (1989). The population over 65 years is 12.1% with infant mortality 8.7. Life expectancy in 1989 was 74.0 years for males and 80.0 years for females.

Cardiovascular disease, cancer and accidents are the main causes of death and morbidity, even though infectious and parasitic diseases still attain a significant level in certain areas and social groups (in many instances linked with deficiencies in the infrastructure of sanitation as well as sociocultural difficulties of access to health services, especially those of health promotion).

Many of the prevalent health problems are related to changes in the environment and personal habits. About 61% of the population do not smoke. Non-alcohol consumers represent 30.1% (17.95% men; 41.3% women). Drug abuse is an increasing problem, associated with AIDS in the case of parenteral use (64% of total declared cases).

Health protection has been a constitutional right since 1978. The National Health System was established by law, in 1986, as the aggregation of different public health agencies (social security, public health, etc) organised in Regional Health Services, coordinated by an Interterritorial Committee and the Ministry of Health. Some 98% of the population is covered by public financed care, mostly provided by public institutions; 10% have private insurance.

In 1991, 66% of public funds came from general taxes and 29.5% from social security fee. Public expenditure in 1990 was 5.3% of GDP, and represented 77.4% of total health expenditure: 64% for specialised care,

32% for PHC (drug prescription included - 20%); 4% other services (management included). Expenditure on health has been growing since 1988 and taking up a larger share of the public health expenditure per capita is about USD465 (1988).

Since 1984, PHC has been involved in a process of reform, from an uncoordinated multi-agency organisation to a model based on integration of all different health functions at local level, in districts and basic health zones. The district is a comprehensive structure including: resources management, public health management and health care delivery to a population of between 40,000 to 100,000 inhabitants in rural areas or 100,000 to 200,000 in urban areas. Every district authority has several basic health zones with health centres and other local units. A multidisciplinary group including managers, general practitioners, paediatricians, nurses, social workers, pharmacists, public health veterinarians, epidemiologists, mental health professionals form PHC teams. Some 54% of total population is covered by such PHC teams, which provide the following services: health care delivery; health promotion; environmental health; health education; mental health.

A general hospital provides specialised care to several districts included in a hospital area. There are also regional hospitals for tertiary care services. in 1988, there were 4.6 beds/1000 inhabitants (3.13/1000 in the public sector). There are strong links between the public health network, universities and other educational institutions, especially in medical and nurse education. Research and development is well established as a specific programme mainly oriented to medical research, although other health sciences have been receiving more attention in recent years.

Evaluating the primary health care reforms

Estaban de Manuel, Jose Maria de la Higuera, Francisco Camino, Olga Solas, Joseba Barroeta, Jesus Rodriguez, Eduardo Briones.

In 1982, Andalucia began an extensive programme to reform PHC services in the region. The aim of the reform was to improve the efficiency and quality of the services through increased attention to prevention of diseases, treatment, rehabilitation and promotion of healthy lifestyles. In order to test out the effect of the reforms a study was conducted in two areas of Andalucia; *Estepa* - where the reforms had been introduced; and *Marchena La Luisana* - where the PHC services remained unchanged. The purpose of the research was to test and assess the perception of the population concerning the impact of the reform of PHC services.

Background

During the late 1970's and early 1980's many countries established reform strategies in their health systems based on the concept of PHC. In Spain the National Health Institute was created as the directive body of health services of the Social Security. The different regions of Spain, if they so wished, were given the right to manage their own health services. Andalucia, in 1982, began an ambitious project to reform the PHC services.

The aim was to improve the quality and efficiency of health services with an emphasis on primary care, the prevention of diseases as well as treatment and rehabilitation and the promotion of healthy lifestyles. At the same time, it tried to guarantee health care for every Andalucian based on the principles of equity, accessibility, continuity, humanitarianism and participation. The strategy for the reform of the health services did not follow a previously prepared overall plan. It has been an emerging process formed by a series of rules, actions and budgets established by different actors following the rules of a 'political market.' It is difficult to separate the planning stages from the implementation stages; the magnitude and importance of each is variable.

The shared existence of a single image of how the PHC services were to be in the future has given coherence to the process. However, it is one thing to agree institutional policy at regional level, it is quite another to generate changes in the system which benefit the community.

Methodology

An assessment has been conducted in two rural areas of the province of Seville with very homogenous demographic and socio-economic characteristics: Estepa and Marchena La Luisiana. In the Estepa area, the reforms of the PHC system were implemented in 1986. In Marchena La Luisiana PHC services were not re-organised and are similar to those existing in Estepa before 1986. It was only after the study was completed that the overall programme of reforms was implemented in Marchena La Luisiana. The study was carried out in two stages: the first to identify the specific components of the evaluation model. The second one a comparison between both areas in order to analyse possible variations in the community and the interrelations associated with PHC services.

A panel of experts was formed by members of the district management team, director, nursing coordinators, epidemiologists and professionals, GPs, nurses, social workers and a local politician, to whom the precedents, aims and methodology of the study were explained. Using a Nominal Group technique, the characteristics of the health system and reform of the PHC are grouped, assessed and identified from the perspective of a district manager. The resulting elements are classified in the services and community subsystems and their interrelations. This model of the health system was the guide for the analysis in the evaluation design (Figure 2).

The study had a quasi-experimental design. The PHC systems of Estepa and Marchena La Luisiana were compared according to subsystem components defined in the first stage. The information sources that were used were management documents, activity memorandums, existing information systems and the information provided by the managers of both areas. A random sample of the population of both sexes, aged 18 years and over, and living in the study areas was drawn up. The sample size for Estepa was 401 persons and 390 for Marchena La Luisiana. People were personally interviewed using a structured questionnaire.

Results

Several changes in the PHC system took place during the study period (1986-1990). Many of these in Estepa occurred as a direct consequence of the reform strategy, whereas in Marchena La Luisiana this was not the case. Space does not permit a detailed discussion of the alterations, thus

Figure 2 : Local system model

Community subsystem		Service subsystem
Health needs	<---Accessibility--->	Health system's context
		Material resources
	<---Accessibility--->	
		Human resources
	<------Quality------>	Decision-making
Socio-economic context		
	<---Participation--->	Planning model
		Organisation
	<---Intersectoral--->	
Community values and attitudes	Collaboration	Control model
		Activities and services

114

only the more notable have been highlighted. One immediate benefit to Estepa of being included in the reform plans was that more resources became available. This resulted in not only more GPs and nurses than before but also the services of a paediatrician, gynaecologist, dentist and mental health team were secured. In Estepa GPs increased from 3.06 to 5.41/10,000 inhabitants whereas in Marchena the rate remained constant at 3.17/10,000. Moreover, Marchena did not have the services of a dentist, radiology technician or physiotherapist. Other changes taking place in Estepa but not Marchena were: introduction of centralised medical records; modification and extension of the role and responsibilities of nurses; preventive services and health promotion programmes were introduced; and doctors hours were increased from 12.5 to 40 hours per week.

In Estepa 82%, and Marchena La Luisiana 77% of the population were born in the same community of residence; the rest have been living in this community for more than 10 years. The demographic structure of both populations has a similar profile. One of every 4 persons living in Estepa or Marchena La Luisiana was young, between 18 to 24 years of age and 17% were older than 65 during the period of study. The average age of both populations was 43 years.

Both populations had a high illiteracy level. Rates of literacy were higher for the women, for those older than 45, and for residents of Marchena La Luisiana (22%) with respect to Estepa (17%). The basic economic activity in the two areas was agriculture. However, there was a more predominant industrial sector in Marchena La Luisiana. This was not reflected in its occupational structure with a larger component of industrial businessmen, manual labourers, and qualified tradesmen. In Estepa, 54% of the occupied population works in agriculture, whereas in Marchena La Luisiana the proportion is only 39%. With respect to the occupational status there existed a relatively low rate of unemployment; 7% in Estepa and 8% in Marchena La Luisiana.

There were no important differences in the attitudes and values of the two populations with respect to the influence of environmental conditions, life styles and the health services on health. However the ill effects of smoking and alcohol were never acknowledged by the Estepa population. Whether this was the effect of health education programmes in the reformed area requires a more in-depth study.

The perceived health status was quite good in both areas. However, there were socio-economical and cultural variables. In spite of the organisational and resource differences between one area and the other, health problems are very similar in both areas. From a medical point of view the changes have been directed towards diagnostic precision and the treatment of acute health problems. Emphasis in prevention was focused on mother and child care, immunisation, food hygiene and environmental sanitation. Most acute and chronic problems (Tables 8 and 9) had an important dimension (headache, depression, allergies and weakness) with which traditional clinical practice seldom dealt.

There was an apparent paradox between perceived health problems and demand for new services (Table 10). The specialists required provide mostly acute medical care, while the majority of the perceived health problems would benefit from services in which the preventive, psychological, and rehabilitative components of care are a significant part. The exception was dental care and emergency services. Centralisation of on-duty medical services after 17.00 in the Estepa health centre, abolished round-the-clock access to GPs in every small village. The feeling that their doctor 'had been taken away', was compensated to some extent by the perception that emergency services had improved (73% of the population).

The percentage of people that used health services was high in both areas (Table 11). As expected, there were no differences between both areas, although the percentage of use of private medical services was almost double in the non reformed area. The highest use of nurses' services and immunisations in Estepa showed a greater emphasis in preventive and caring services.

The level of satisfaction with accessibility was high (Table 12). Respondents were satisfied with the centres hours of service and they did not find it difficult to get access to a doctor. However, people were not satisfied with the time they spent in waiting rooms when they attended their GPs' offices.

Family doctors were more highly valued in the reformed area; 61% of the Estepa population preferred a GP over a specialist. The preferences were inverted in the smaller villages, and in the non-reformed area where more than 60% of the population preferred a specialist.

People trusted their doctors. Again, the score was higher in Estepa. Although 74% of those surveyed thought they were better looked after when they paid for the service, only 21% preferred a private doctor to a public one. The image of the health centres was good; 60% of the Marchena population would rather have more health centres than hospitals.

Satisfaction with quality of services was not easy to assess, and further statistical analysis may provide a clearer understanding of the elements

116

Table 8
Estimated prevalence of 'acute' problems in the two areas

Estepa	Frequency %	Marchena-la Luisiana	Frequency %
Respiratory	37.4	Respiratory	30.3
Headache	25.4	Headache	24.1
Weakness	11.2	Toothache	12.8
Edema	7.7	Weakness	11.8
Gastritis	7.5	Gastritis	8.5
Toothache	6.7	Edema	8.5
Fever	6.5	Conjunctivitis	6.7
Conjunctivitis	3.7	Fever	6.4
Cystitis	2.7	Cystitis	5.4
Palpitations	2.5	Vomiting	4.1

Table 9
Estimated prevalence of 'chronic' problems in the two areas

Estepa	Frequency %	Marchena-la Luisiana	Frequency %
Caries	70.3	Caries	62.3
Arthritis	41.1	Arthritis	42.3
Headache	33.9	Headache	37.2
Arteriosclerosis	27.4	Arteriosclerosis	23.6
Depression	21.7	Depression	21.0
Hypertension	19.7	Haemorrhoids	20.0
Haemorrhoids	19.2	Hypertension	19.0
Anaemia	16.7	Constipation	18.7
Allergies	14.5	Weakness	16.2
Varicose Veins	13.7	Allergies	15.6

Table 10
Health services public say are needed

	Estepa		Marchena-la Luisiana
1	Emergency services	1	Cardiologist
2	Paediatrician	2	Paediatrician
3	Traumatologist	3	Traumatologist
4	Ophthalmologist	4	Dentist
5	Cardiologist	5	Gynaecologist
6	Gynaecologist	6	Radiologist
7	Dentist	7	Ophthalmologist
8	Radiologist	8	Emergency services
9	Radiologist	9	Hospital beds
10	Hospital beds	10	More G.P.'s

Table 11
Use of the health services

Health services	Estepa	Health services	Marchena-la Luisiana
General Practice	85.8	General Practice	70.8
Pharmacist	79.1	Pharmacist	61.3
Nurse	71.3	Nurse	57.2
Tests	53.6	Tests	44.9
Immunisations	46.1	Immunisations	38.7
Emergency service	25.9	Dentist	31.0
Dentist	25.4	Emergency service	30.3
Radiology	13.7	Veterinarian	10.8
Veterinarian	9.5	Paediatrician	10.6
Paediatrician	4.5	Radiology	4.7
Gynaecologist	3.0	Ophthalmologist	5.6

Table 12
Accessibility of the services (% satisfied)

	Estepa	Rest	Marchena	La Lusiana
Distance to be covered to set to the centre	61.0	89.0	78.6	86.0
Timetable open to patients	74.4	66.9	69.4	71.3
Waiting time before entering the surgery	21.8	31.1	27.3	43.0
It is easy and comfortable to see the doctor when necessary	76.5	68.7	65.5	69.8

119

and relations of consumer satisfaction. More than 75% of those who took part in the survey stated that the overall quality of the services of PHC in the past three years had improved. However, there were important differences between both areas and Estepa village, where the new centre was built and where the majority of the services were situated. In fact, 73% of those who took part in the survey in both areas considered that the emergency services were better, a percentage which increased to almost 90% in Estepa village as compared with 61% for the rest of the Estepa area.

Although the overall level of satisfaction with quality of the services was very similar in both areas, there were obvious differences in the appreciation of concrete aspects of the structure of health services and the process of care. For example, the percentage of those who were satisfied with the treatment received from the medical personnel and from the nurses and with the time dedicated to each patient was greater in Estepa.

Conclusion

The health system on a local level is a complex entity made up of a multitude of elements and people with different objectives, necessities, values and behaviours. A change in any one of them has effects on the others. The assessment of the PHC reform was not easy. It was necessary to simplify the reality to be able to describe it, to establish comparisons and to interpret them. The isolated analysis of each element would be easier (less complex) but biased.

However, considering the whole health system, including the community sub-system and comparing the reformed and non-reformed areas enabled a better understanding of the effect of the changes, and to generate explanatory hypothesis for further investigation.

The changes in the services affected the structure and organisation of the system. Though the changes were supposed to be implemented in the whole area of Estepa, the effects of the health services reforms were mostly perceived in the main town. The perceptions of the inhabitants of the smaller villages were very similar to those of the non-reformed areas.

New policy strategies that deal with the patient professional-relation, preventive and caring services, and with the image of the system are needed. Incentives for professionals and continuing education should be emphasised, while continuing the development of better facilities, health care organisation, and budget and human resources administration. An explicit external marketing policy should certainly render good benefits too.

Reducing inequalities for pregnant women by means of primary health care

Joan Puig, Jose Salazar and Concha Colomer

This study compares the prenatal care given to women under a new primary health care delivery model and under a traditional model. Access to and use of services are evaluated. The effect of the new system in reducing inequalities was also assessed.

This study was carried out in the 01 Health Area of the Valencian Community. This area, situated in the north of the Community, consists of the natural regions of El Baix Maestrat and Els Port de Morella and has a population of 63,474 people living in the two coastal towns and the remaining small, widely scattered villages. Out of the total of 12,012 women (aged 15-44) living in this area, 8,217 (68%), live in the coastal zone, covered by the new PHC model and have access to a prenatal health care programme and the possibility of contacting a PHC team; while the rest, 3,795 (32.59%) inhabit rural zones in the interior.

In the new model, midwives carry out a prenatal care programme. They use a standard protocol that includes a specified number of consultations and anciliary tests, childbirth preparation sessions, the completion of a case history and record book on the pregnant woman (the latter is kept by the woman) and precise guidelines about referral requirements. Women not covered by this programme are cared for by a national health service obstetrician, or by private doctors in or outside the Health Area. The only referral maternity clinic is in the General Hospital at Castellon, 70 km away.

Methodology

All the women who had just had a child were interviewed personally during the period 15 May 1990 to 15 August 1990. Most interviews were conducted at the referral hospital and, when that was not possible, at the woman's home. All interviews were carried out within 30 days of delivery. Information was collected on: the access to and use of services; the type of provider; motivation for choosing that type of provider; Care activities; and background and socio-economic status.

The women were classified as 'exposed' if they lived in a basic health area or in a town where the new model has been implemented (implying the existence of a midwife who is carrying out the programme activities and the existence of a PHC team), and as 'unexposed' if they lived in traditional health care areas.

The technique used to evaluate the existing differences between levels was the non-parametric Mann Whitney (Olds *et al*., 1986), due to the ordinal measurement scale, the unusual distribution of variables such as the age and time taken in accessing the services, and the number of observations. The 2 x 2 tables were evaluated with the Chi square using the Yates correction. In order to make comparisons between socioeconomic levels, two levels (middle-high, and middle-low) were constructed by means of cluster analysis using socioeconomic variables (income, occupational status and educational level).

Results

A total of 100 women were interviewed after childbirth: 80% were exposed and 20% were unexposed. Both populations were similar in respect to: average age (27 for exposed women and 28 for unexposed women); the number of children (1.8 for exposed women and 1.45 for unexposed women); level of education, income and occupation. Similarity, the groups did not differ with regard to partner's income, educational level or occupational status.

Of those women who used the new model, 36% went to the clinic on foot, 43% went in their own vehicle, and one percent used public transport. In contrast, women who used the traditional model (unexposed) mainly drove their own cars to clinic appointments (90%). There was a statistically significant difference in mode of transport used between groups to attend prenatal appointments ($p < 0.00001$).

The average travel time from home to clinics was 15 minutes for those enrolled in the new model and 46 for those enrolled in the traditional model ($p < 0.00001$).

There were no statistically significant differences between the groups in their perceptions of the convenience of clinic schedules. Fewer women receiving care under the new model thought their mode of transport inconvenient compared with their counterparts receiving traditional care. Nearly a quarter of both groups felt clinic schedules were inconvenient.

The women were asked if they had participated in childbirth preparation activities. Only two women enrolled in the traditional model did some kind of childbirth preparation activity. Out of the 80 women exposed to the new PCH model, 37 (46%) received childbirth preparation. The differences between exposed and unexposed populations were statistically significant (P<0.02).

Two socioeconomic stratas, middle-low and middle-high, were constructed by means of cluster analysis. The middle-low strata consisted of 66 women, and the middle-high of 31; there was not sufficient information for grouping three women (68% and 70%) from middle-low (Table 13).

Whereas 21 (40%) out of 52 exposed women from middle-low strata used childbirth preparation services, none of the 14 unexposed women from the same socio-economic level used or has access to these services. Sixteen (64%) out of the 25 exposed women from middle-high status used childbirth preparation services versus two (33%) out of six middle-high unexposed women who also had access to this kind of service.

Exposed women, as a group, used childbirth preparations services more than unexposed women (48% versus 10%). But when we observed the pattern of use between the two socioeconomic groups of exposed women (Table 13), the percentage of women from the middle-high status using these services was higher (P=0.0071).

The women were also asked to indicate their motives for use of the services and relative influence on their decision making of each motive. Answers were graded on an ordinal scale (1, great influence to 5, no influence). Women mainly answered that if they went to the midwife it was because they had no other choice (83.6%) (Table 14). Although the availability of childbirth preparation activities was a major influence for 53% of the women, this high percentage was mostly due to the middle-high socioeconomic exposed women who went to a private sector obstetrician (data not shown), and used the facilities provided by the programme in the public sector.

Conclusion

The new model was effective in promoting the use of prenatal care services among the exposed population, (at least 37 women of the 80 exposed pursued childbirth preparation exercises). The effectiveness of the new model can be quantified: 46% of the exposed population were covered.

However, when the socio-economic component is added, the new model is no more accessible than the old one for women of middle-low socio-economic level. The use of prenatal care by these women is significantly lower, and the prenatal care offered by the new model was used more intensively by women from the middle-high sector. This highlights a phenomenon described as the inverse prevention law (Silvestre *et al*,

Table 13
Use of services by exposure and socioeconomic level

Child birth preparation sessions	Exposed Middle low	Middle high	Unexposed Middle low	Middle high	Total
Yes	21	16	0	2	39
No	31	9	14	4	58
Total	52	25	14	6	97

Table 14
Motivations to use midwife services among exposed population (percentage)

Motivations	Influence Major	Not at all
Convenient schedule	12.7	81.9
Knew the midwife	18.2	76.3
Preparation for childbirth	52.8	40.0
Gave more time	11.0	81.8
No other choice	83.6	10.9
Good reports on midwife	29.1	61.8
Aspect of the clinic	5.5	89.1
Took little time to get there	10.9	81.0
Good technical resources	16.4	69.1
Could not afford a private service	3.6	94.6
Against private health care	1.8	96.3
Free health care	9.1	89.1
Previous pregnancies	11.0	85.5

1990), where health promoting activities do not reach the whole social spectrum with the same intensity, and those that are supposed to be more in need of these activities because of their socioeconomic status, are the ones that benefit less.

On the evidence presented it can be concluded that the new health care model based on PHC, is effective in improving accessibility and the use of prenatal services in the exposed population. However, on the question of the equity of the system (both social and geographical) this requires an in depth study on strategies peculiar to it in order to overcome the present limitations.

Sweden

Primary health care

By international standards, health in Sweden is relatively good. Infant mortality is low, at about 5.9 deaths per 1,000 in the first year of life. Average life expectancy is 74.1 years for males and 80.1 years for females. Just as in other advances industrialised countries, health problems in Sweden are related not so much to infections and under-nutrition as to environment and life-style.

The predominant diseases are cardiovascular conditions and cancer. The proportion of senior citizens has increased, with almost 17% of the population currently 65 or over. The incidence of disease and injury varies between different social groups. Certain occupational categories, low income groups, the unemployed, single people, and immigrants encounter greater health hazards than others.

Health and medical care are regarded as an important part of the Swedish welfare system. Its fundamental principle is that all citizens are entitled to good health and equal access to health and medical care, regardless of where they live and their economic circumstances. In line with this principle, health and medical care are seen as a public sector responsibility which is supported by a national health insurance system. In 1985, Parliament laid down certain guidelines for future health services and medical policy. These guidelines include:

* An improvement in the general standard of health should be achieved, implying a continuing active and coordinated health care policy which must concentrate on eliminating health risks. Care on equal terms for the entire population must be ensured.

*   Health and medical care should be administered primarily within
        the public service sector and should be based on public
        responsibility, collective financing, proximity, accessibility and
        freedom of choice.

Responsibility for health and medical care, is a duty of the 23 county
councils and three large municipalities. These units, with populations
ranging from some 300,000 to 1.5 million, also operate the public dental
and mental health services. Responsibility for social welfare services and
environmental hygiene rests primarily with the municipalities, which
currently number 284 and have populations ranging from about 5,000 to
700,000. Private health care exists but on a limited scale.

There are approximately 13.6 hospital beds in Sweden per 1,000
inhabitants. There are also around seven places per 1,000 inhabitants in
municipal homes for the elderly. In contrast, the number of out-patient
visits to physicians is comparatively low - about three visits per inhabitant
per year. In addition there are around two visits to district nurses and one
visit for paramedical care. Outpatient care is organised into primary care
districts. Each district which assumes primary responsibility for the health
of the population in its area has one or more local health care centres and
at least one nursing home for long-term care.

Efforts are being made to enable the ill and disabled to be cared for at
home as much as possible. Nursing staff of the primary care services and
municipally employed social welfare personnel work together in teams.
Occasionally, when primary care resources are insufficient for diagnosis
or treatment, responsibility may be transferred to the county or regional
level medical care services.

Health and medical care costs have increased very rapidly in recent
decades, climbing during the past 15 years by 15-20% annually in current
prices. Today they amount to 9.2% of GNP. Health and medical care is
financed primarily by income taxes levied by the county councils.
Distribution of health and medical care costs are as follows: Somatic
short-term care 48%; Somatic long-term care 24%; Outpatient primary
care 16%; Psychiatric care 12%.

To strengthen confidence in PHC by changing the communication interface between PHC, the hospital and the patients

Bertil Marklund and Henric Hultin

Swedish health services are heavily reliant on hospital services. In attempts to 'Tip the Balance towards Primary Health Care', it is crucial to strengthen the confidence in PHC. This project shows that it is possible to act as one health care organisation without encountering demarcation difficulties between PHC and the hospital.

Alvsborg County is located in the south-west of Sweden. It has 430,000 residents, which makes the County Council the fourth largest in the country. It is the most industrialised county in Sweden. The County Council is responsible for health and medical services, care of the mentally retarded, education for agriculture, forestry and nursing services, and the administration of tourism, enterprise and cultural amenities. The State County Administration and County Council have their headquarters in the old county town of Vanersborg. Each municipality has its own administration.

The PHC in the County Council is organised in 10 separate districts each with its own political board (subordinate to the Executive Committee of the County Council). Hospital care is organised in two districts with their political boards: one for the northern and one for the southern part of the county. Almost all of the health care services and institutions are owned, run and funded by the County Council. The County Council has a rather decentralised organisational structure. Within yearly budgets and master plans, the local boards have freedom to run their organisation as they see fit. Also, inside the district organisation, daily decision-making is decentralised, mostly to the heads of clinical departments and health centres. Locally there is considerable cooperation between the social welfare and health services in PHC, both at the city-district level and at the local level.

The area specially studied in this subproject is the Vanersborg-Trollhattan area. In this area with about 90,000 inhabitants there are two cities, 15 km apart: Vanersborg and Trollhattan. In Vanersborg their are few immigrants but in Trollhattan there are many, especially in the metal industries where there are a lot of Finnish-speaking employees. There are about 50 different languages spoken amongst the inhabitants. The unemployment rate is low compared with the rest of the country (although rising since 1990).

The overall health situation can be characterised by the mortality for males 0-64 years of age. For both cities, it is less than the national average. The industrial city of Trollhattan has a lot of alcohol-related problems and some problems with ethnic isolation and language difficulties.

The city of Vanersborg has three health centres with different catchment areas (in the rural surroundings there is another one). There are district nurses, who are engaged in home care but who also have a clinic base. There are two general long term care homes and one for psychiatric long term care. Facilities for day care are also available. There is thorough preventive care for pregnant women and small children. PHC in Trollhattan is organised in a corresponding way. There are four health centres in the city.

Until the beginning of 1988, there had been a general hospital in each city, of which the one in Vanersborg was the most specialised. In January 1988, a brand new hospital (in Trollhattan, but close to the border of Vanersborg) was opened which replaced the two older ones. The new hospital serves all of the northern part of the county (170,000 inhabitants) as did the other two hospitals before.

Previously the PHC emergency unit providing evening, night and weekend service in the two cities and surrounding rural areas was in the centre of Trollhattan. As of January 1988, the service has been united with new general hospital. Agreements on allocation of the duties of care at the joint emergency unit were prepared in conjunction with this project

Aim of the project

The aim of this project is to strengthen confidence and trust in primary health care on the part of the population and promote better utilisation of resources. This was accomplished by giving patients simple and concordant information about where to obtain care for their problems; and by taking care of the patient at the appropriate level of care system.

It is desirable that patients experience PHC and hospital as one health care organisation, without encountering 'border' difficulties. This requires adequate medical guidelines for referral and reassuring treatment during the whole episode of care.

Activities and methods

An activity of the programme to strengthen PHC was to emphasise the role of PHC-nurses in advising and referring patients. In order to facilitate their work and also to support the coordination of the PHC and hospital activities, work started with the development of teaching material and a tool for telephone counselling.

A questionnaire for each of the most common reasons for seeking contact with medical services (Marklund *et al*, 1989a) was developed. The questionnaires were designed as 'trees' with even more specific questions and preliminary decisions to be used as a basis for the advice given to the patient during telephone contacts. These 'trees' (Figure 3) were designed in collaboration between PHC physicians and the hospital specialists. The 'trees' also were expected to illustrate how and where the patients with the symptoms described will get the best care (Marklund *et al.*, 1990).

The PHC nurses, responsible for information and telephone counselling in the health centres wentthrough an educational programme using the questionnaire as teaching material. The feasibility of the questionnaire both as teaching material and as an instrument in giving patients medical advices was tested at one health centre (Marklund *et al*, 1989b). Evaluation showed that the quality of advice improved and that confidence and satisfaction with the work also increased among the participating nurses. A follow up by letter was undertaken in Autumn 1987 to ascertain their satisfaction with the advice and care received. The vast majority of patients were satisfied with changes introduced in the new system.

In order to achieve that patients would have similar answers and reactions from the hospital emergency nurses as from the PHC nurses, the same educational programme was carried out with them. The hospital doctors involved in the emergency unit were active in the programme. The same follow up of the proper use of the questionnaire 'tree' and of the satisfaction of the patients has been done after the educational programme was completed. During five weeks, all telephone calls from patients with acute illnesses were registered at the emergency unit (200 patients). The patients were predominantly positive to the telephone counselling with nurses, and the majority were satisfied with the nurses way of doing the counselling.

The number of ambulatory patients to the health centres and the hospital units was studied during a period of three months before the move into the new joint hospital, and compared with a corresponding period after the move. The result was that the number of visits to health centres in Vanesborg and Trollhattan has increased, and the number of visits to the hospital has decreased correspondingly (about 10%).

Figure 3 : Flow chart for 'cough' among adults with no fever

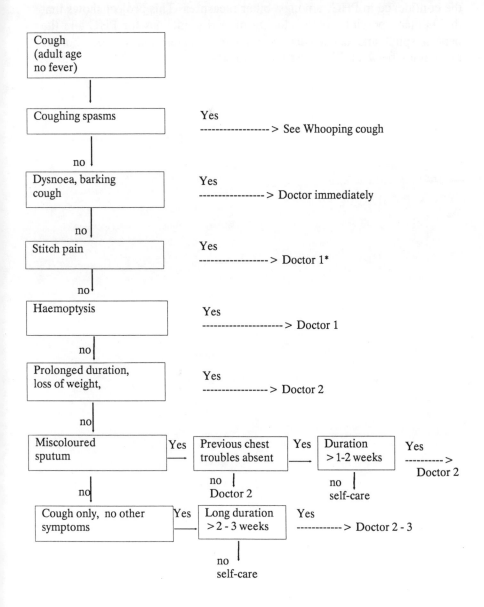

* (1 signifies appointment with the doctor the same day, 2 = one week, 3 = three weeks)

131

Conclusion

To tip the balance towards primary health care, it is crucial to strengthen the confidence in PHC, amongst other measures. This project shows that this is made possible by developing mutual guidelines for PHC and the near hospital and act as one health care organisation without border difficulties between PHC and the hospital.

Blekinge County Council projects

Blekinge County contributed two projects to 'Tipping the Balance Towards Primary Health Care'. The first one involved the creation of study circles to educate and promote behaviour change for coronary risk reduction. The study circles, instead of being expert led, were consumer led and used professionals only as resource persons. The second project was designed to improve primary prevention through opportunistic PHC screening. Both projects were seen as good examples of health promotion and targeted intervention. During the TTB-Project, a number of unintended effects and 'spin-off' effects were observed.

Encouraged by the results of the second project, the Board of Blekinge County Council in 1989 set targets for prevention of cardiovascular diseases to be achieved through health promotion activities (project one), and behavioural change in the population, complemented by opportunistic screening (project two). The primary target was to reduce myocardial infarct mortality by 15% by the year 2000 through:

* a 4% reduction of blood cholesterol level among the adult population;
* a 2% reduction of the diastolic blood pressure among the adult population; and
* a 25% reduction of the number of smokers in the population.

The development of the projects has resulted in increased cooperation between PHC and the Department of Internal Medicine of the Karlskrona Hospital, increased skills in PHC about rehabilitation after acute infarction, and increased skills among PHC staff about nutrition.

Similarly, the process of developing the preventive skills in PHC also has also led to cooperation between PHC districts in Blekinge and the Regional University Hospital in Lund/Malmo. Scientific studies based on the initiatives in Blekinge are beginning to emerge from this cooperation. Finally, the identification and analysis of health problems, the formulation of a strategy at various levels and the implementation of that strategy cooperatively has given to all involved experience which makes them better equipped to meet other challenges in the health field.

Background

Blekinge is located in the south-east of Sweden. It has 150,000 inhabitants, which makes the County one of the smallest in the country, both in area and population. It has five municipalities and is divided into two main health districts. Due to both migration and a birth rate lower than the death rate, there has been a diminishing population since the 1970's. The proportion in the age group 25-64 years is smaller and the proportion over 65 years of age is slightly higher than in the country as a whole. Blekinge has a very low proportion of immigrants to support population growth.

There is a relatively high population density in the county. Unemployment is higher than in the country in general, especially for youth and women. Industrial production is the mainstay of the economy and employes 34% of the population. The public sector is almost as large but mainly in child care and nursing and dominated by women. The mean-income is lower than in the country as a whole, and so is the disposable income for families with children. Municipal taxes are comparatively high and so are the living costs for the 'typical family'.

The inhabitants generally show lower morbidity and mortality than the country as a whole. They also consume less health care. One of the most apparent deviations is a higher mortality in heart diseases compared with the rest of southern part of the country. Regarding general health indicators, the County has comparatively high rates of sickness, especially work related, and pensions (prior to 65 years of age). Social care in terms of aid to retired is well developed and so is paediatric nursing.

Coronary Heart Disease (CHD) is the leading cause of death in Sweden today, especially among men 45-64 years of age. About 40% of CHD deaths are due to myocardial infarction. In March 1987, a report on leading causes of death in the southern region of Sweden during 1979-1984, showed an increase in mortality in acute myocardial infarction in Blekinge of approximately 40%, among men and women, in the ages 1-64 years, compared to the average level of the region. A calculation of so called 'lost years' shows that tjere is excess CHD mortality among the younger adults.

This report led to the decision to take action against ischemic heart disease within the frame of the TTB-Project. During the last few years, it has been fully recognised in Blekinge that prevention of ischemic heart disease demands a community strategy in combination with a medical one. Therefore, participation in the TTB-project was concentrated around the following two projects.

Health promotion through discussion with the general public

Lars-Olof Ljunberg

Aim of the project

This was an initiative to start a broad political dialogue on health with the general public. The interest of the public and different associations are valuable resources in the work for better public health. The connections with local needs and circumstances were underlined in the material that was discussed. The view collected through the contacts are basic to resource planning and preventive measures in the future both locally and regionally.

Through the County's unit for community and environmental health, information was compiled regarding environments, health situations and living conditions. On this basis, a book was written on eight themes of importance for future public health: new perspectives; new diseases; public health and social structure; environmental pollution; accident risks; health and life-styles; social life and care; and resources for health. The book was seen as the starting point for discussions about the local situation. The aim was to make possible exchanges of experiences about the local conditions. It was not a study of the art of how to manage personal health. So experts were not necessary.

Co-operation between Blekinge County Council and Blekinge County Study Association led to the start of study circles in all municipalities and in local study associations; approximately 130 circles and 1,500 persons (1 % of the population) participated in the discussions. In the same way, all employees in the hospitals and PHC had the opportunity to join study circles during working-time in order to exchange experiences. The County Council paid all costs of production and distribution of the books. Participants paid no fees to take part.

The members of a circle could shift the responsibility for the meetings according to their interest. They assembled further material from newspapers and other sources to throw light on the subject. As support, they were able to ask anyone of 150 'resource-persons' from a list of politicians and experts which the County Council has asked to participate if the groups so wish. Eight meetings, of about three hours each, were carried out. The number of meetings often increased when a subject was regarded as being especially interesting by the group. Visits to places or institutions were often arranged and contacts were made between different groups and associations.

Scenarios and new dialogue

The members of a circle summed up their discussions about each theme in a short scenario about the future and what they believed was important to do to change the direction of events. The scenario or summaries from the circles were compiled and published by the County Council, so all participants learn about each others views and opinions. A new discussion could then start. A local health plan was written on the basis of the suggestions and reactions from the public. Such a plan would then be implemented in full co-operation and co-ordinated action together with the local inhabitants.

Branches of the process

The process discussed above had many facets. Municipalities, political organisations, public associations and individuals have made arrangements and actions within the frames of the project. Several local environmental problems were brought up and, in some cases, actions taken to solve them on initiative from the circles. Co-operation and channelling has begun of the widespread engagement for better environment and public health.

This movement in the future will become self-sustaining and health problems will feature in discussions about environment and living conditions, as people find out that their views are valued. Furthermore, action will be taken on different social levels and on initiatives from many groups.

New strategies in public health

The County Council took an important step in line with WHO principles to renew the methods for better public health. Basic facts and proposals for health-political discussions were presented. The general public was deeply interested in health matters and many persons were ready to take part in preventive actions and improving public health. To find ways to reach as many of their inhabitants as possible and find methods to gain and use their engagement was not so easy.

The County Council decided to revise the study material and to present an up-dated version during the Spring 1991. During the Autumn 1991 new study circles started, this time in cooperation with a number of trade unions. It was assumed that discussions about new diseases, public health and social structures and health and lifestyles would increase awareness among the general public of the risk factors for ischemic heart disease and therefore promoter healthier life-styles.

Primary prevention of cardiac and arterial disease by opportunistic screening

Lars-Olof Ljunberg

Aim of the project

The prevention of heart disease through PHC has been thoroughly discussed during the last decade. Opportunistic screening complementing some form of population strategy was recommended. A substantial proportion of the population visits general practitioners within a certain span of time, therefore, it is hardly possible to expect the general practitioner to do this kind of screening unaided. This study demonstrated the feasibility of an opportunistic screening or case-finding model in general practice, with the physician as initiator controlling the inclusion rate and the nurse and nurse-aid responsible for the follow-up management, without any extra resources. The study included all 25-29 year old residents of four of the five parishes in the Lyckeby area (n=6657).

Methodology

The physicians at the Lyckeby PHC Center in Blekinge (16,000 inhabitants) use in their routine practice, established techniques for blood pressure measurement and hypertension diagnoses. In individuals, 25-29 years, blood pressure measurement was followed by an evaluation of smoking habits and determination of blood cholesterol. Individuals, with a diastolic blood pressure > 90 or blood cholesterol > 6.9 mmol/1 or smoking habits were considered to be at increased risk for cardiovascular disease and in need of risk factor intervention and follow-up. Non-pharmacological and pharmacological treatment of hypertension was given according to the norms of the Swedish Society of Hypertension. For reduction of blood cholesterol, a lipid reducing diet was recommended and smokers were offered help in quitting.

Results

During the first three years of the study, 1,778 patients were included, or 27% of the total population at risk. Among patients 40-59 years old, the proportion of those who visited the PHC centre of Lyekeby was 49% for men and 46% for women. The lowering of serum-cholesterol after two years was 6.4% for men between 40 and 59 years. This follow-up included all patients, even those with low or normal risk factors. The compliance to the follow up differed according to age and risk group.

Conclusion

This study demonstrated the feasibility of undertaking multiple cardiovascular risk factor intervention in PHC with resources presently used for hypertension management. The results also indicate that a substantial proportion of the population at risk will be detected. The study continues.

Monitoring of primary health care

Hans Ekman

The project set out to develop and implement a more effective method to monitor PHC. It was undertaken on the assumption that an integrated monitoring of resource usage, performance and goal achievement, based on systematic use of comparisons not only would improve PHC monitoring but also create incentives for the development of adequate performance measurements and goal targets. Further aims were to support the continuing decentralisation of decision-making and responsibilities, and facilitate the task of meeting increased demand of a growing number of elderly within restricted financial resources.

Background

Bohus County Council is located on the west coast of Sweden. The County has 305,000 inhabitants of whom 16% are 65 years or older. Traditionally, employment has been in farming, fishing, forestry and shipyards to which refining and other activities have now been added. Within the County there are 14 PHC Boards which have responsibility for primary health care in their areas, and serve populations ranging from 9,000 to 50,000. The boundaries of the 14 primary health care areas coincide with those of the 14 local communes, who have responsibility for schools, social services, physical planning, and so on.

The project originated in a debate within the county about whether or not the current method of resource allocation took proper account of needs in various PHC areas. This led to a demand for intensified monitoring to try to assess what are the effects of the alleged relative lack of resources in certain areas.

Methodology

The thrust of the project was to change the process and usage of monitoring rather than to introduce specific measurements. A working group of economists and planners developed the indicators which were based on the information already available. The new presentation of the information, which tried to integrate resource usage and activities, was influenced by a small number of planners who had grown increasingly frustrated with the lack of monitoring of the impact of decision-making.

The initial assumption about changes to the monitoring process was discussed in several groups, for instance, GP's steering committee, PHC managers, and a special one-day seminar about monitoring with about 100 participants. After the initial presentation of the new monitoring information, several meetings were held at PHC local level. These activities helped in creating limited but not absolute acceptance of the methods.

The purpose of the project was to assess whether or not changes introduced in monitoring PHC improved its effectiveness. This study concentrated more on process analysis, rather than on the advantages/disadvantages of using certain specific measurements/indicators. The four changes introduced through the monitoring process were:

* Integration of monitoring of resource usage, activities and goal achievement;
* Systematically use of comparisons;

* Integration of the monitoring process with that of planning and budgeting;
* Presentation of the monitoring information.

These changes were implemented during the three years 1988-90. Three reports were produced for each year which compared in slightly different ways, the subactivities of the 14 PHC areas. These reports and the monitoring process were presented and discussed at various meetings with managers, providers, and politicians.

Results

Resource allocation in the county attempts to be needs-based. The allocation of resources to PHC boards was based on a comparison in each district between population needs to be met by services and available resources; a modified RAWP-type formula. The proxy indicator of need was population utilisation of each of the four groups of service (GP services; care of the elderly; prevention; and rehabilitation, including physiotherapy). The population was divided into groups according to age and sex. The estimated relative need for the population in each PHC area in each group of service was weighted according to the groups percentage of total costs.

The indicators to test whether or not a needs-based form of resource allocation was effective were:

* number of visits (G.P.s and other health care workers), separately per inhabitant, in each PHC area, as compared to the county average after adjustment for age and sex;

* number of in-patient days in nursing homes, number of admissions to these homes and number of patients in home care of the elderly;

* costs per inhabitant for each service, after age and sex adjustment, as compared to the county average.

The project increased the interest in monitoring. The new monitoring process, which subdivided PHC activities, was much closer to the individual health care worker. For instance, when comparing physiotherapy in a small PHC area there might only be two individuals involved.

Health care workers interest was manifested in two ways, by questioning the figures presented, and the measurements used. The feedback of monitoring information, in a more understandable form than before, to those responsible for services created an awareness of the importance to report accurate figures in the standardised statistical returns which have been in use for many years in the country. When monitoring becomes more than a set of statistical tables, the debate becomes more intense about the reliability and validity of the measurements in use. One outcome has been that some groups of health workers began to explore possible alternative measurements.

The project also led to a debate about definitions of the various measurements used in health care monitoring in the county. As a result, the planning department issued a revised set of definitions of measurements, which were based on national standards. However, in at least two instances, the project suggested the need for changes to the national standards. The project activities also led to a greater awareness of the necessity for improved information about the patient visits to health care workers, as previously, only the number of visits were included in the standard statistical returns. It was suggested that information on age, sex, domicile of the patient, and reason for the visit should be included in the continuous data collection, because although in-patient care registers record this kind of information, out-patient records did not.

Two of the aims of the project were to assist in decisions about the allocation of resources between different PHC sub-activities, and to identify areas of low productivity. During the first year, the county used the new monitoring information to raise questions with the local boards about productivity and allocation policy. This led to heated arguments in some instances. The traditionally very independent PHC boards were not used to be questioned in this way. As a consequence, the distribution of the monitoring information changed in the second year: only very general information was included in the annual report to the county council and the centre did not raise questions with the local level. The detailed information concerning each PHC area with comparisons with the county average was sent directly to each PHC board.

The presentation of the monitoring information was difficult to explain to politicians and managers, many of whom were unfamiliar with some of the techniques. For example, monitoring was hampered by the 'budget perspective' (whether the budget limit was exceeded or not), instead of concentrating on productivity, quality and effectiveness. A major negative development was the increasingly lack of resources, which caused reorientation of activities and led to lay-offs of personnel. As a result, major organisational reforms are now under way but these are taking a lot of the time of managers and central planners.

Conclusion

Although the project was not as successful as had been hoped, there are a number of points on which it is worth commenting. They serve as a starting point for discussions about how to achieve effective monitoring.

Much more effort is needed to find a proper monitoring process linked with the planning and allocating process. The problem is not to create an information system but to know how to use it. Moreover, monitoring cannot be an effective support to decision-making without the support of the decision-makers. Monitoring information might have to be broken down to the level of individual decision-makers (for instance specialists) to become truly effective. Monitoring methods and measurements must be agreed upon at the same time as targets and objectives are set or priority groups identified, and special attention must be given to the purposes of monitoring: for example what questions should monitoring attempt to answer?

Financial initiatives aimed at increasing effectiveness, productivity, quality or similar aspects of health care activity will not automatically ensure more effective monitoring, it must liberate itself from a restricted budget perspective and be more concerned with actual development. Cooperation between different personnel categories should be encouraged and supported.

Monitoring must attempt to integrate information about what has been done (activity); what resources have been used (costs, personnel, building space occupied,); and the quality of care and the outcomes. Monitoring information is difficult to analyse without this integration.

Jamtland County Council projects

The County of Jamtland contributed two projects to 'Tipping the Balance Towards Primary Health Care'. The first one concerned indicators for resource allocation and monitoring, and was aimed at implementing goal-oriented planning and needs-based budgeting. The other project was community participation through the provision of local health boards in PHC.

The County of Jamtland is situated in the centre of Sweden, covering a vast area, and with a population of 135,000, (of which 21% are over 65 years). Population density is low with only three inhabitants/Km., of which 50% is concentrated in the central part of the county. Traditionally, employment has been in farming and forestry, but tourism is growing in importance. In the Ostersund area there are modern industries, such as electronics factories, as well as administrative and educational institutions. Development of health and medical care services has been based on the County Council PHC strategy that follows these principles: primary responsibility regarding public health within the area; democratic policymaking - community participation; decentralised organisation; cooperation (social services, hospital services); comprehensive view of patients and of the organisation; and, accessibility and continuity of care.

PHC and social services areas coincide with those of municipalities. There are eight PHC boards with independent responsibility for activities and budget of the services in their area. The PHC resources include 30 health centres with integrated service; eight health centres in Ostersund; 15 nursing homes (744 beds); and continuous home care. However, nursing homes and some of the home nursing services, will be transferred to the municipal authorities and integrated into the social services. This means that 60 percent of the PHC budget will be transferred as well. This is a major change both within the PHC sector and the social sector. Hospital services are concentrated in one general hospital for medical, psychiatric and geriatric care. Each of the two TTB projects is now discussed in detail.

Planning and budgeting of PHC

*Anne-Marie Jaarnek, Kaj Norrby,
Bo Stencrantz and James Winoy*

Aims of the project

The project sought to develop a new resource allocation process based on the population health needs and to achieve greater efficiency through better monitoring. This project worked on development of the following strategy:

* Goal-oriented planning and health policy making according to the strategy of Health for All;
* Needs-based budgeting;
* Monitoring what and how has been carried out, in terms of quantity, quality and costs; as well of the results, in terms of improved health gains and quality of life, and reduced morbidity and health services demand;
* Local democracy and community participation.

During the period from 1950 to 1985, health services in Sweden experienced a period of expansion in almost all fields. The Swedish system has been, and still is, rather acute care oriented. Central management used fixed norms for resource allocation which did not facilitate adjusting health services to local situations. Since 1985, decentralisation and goal-oriented planning have been an important strategy in Jamtland, as a means to improving efficiency and responsiveness to local needs. This means that a new management philosophy had to be developed, based on management by objectives, needs based budgeting and monitoring by indicators.

There are two main assumptions which underping the work: first, that there cannot be development of planning and budgeting without the related aim of equity; and second, that there must be a decentralisation of resources and power to achieve local goals.

Tipping the balance towards PHC in Jamtlands has been executed through adjusting the budget to the population need for health services; adjusting activities to goals and objectives; and, using indicators to monitor the quality and quantity of PHC services in accordance with stated goals and objectives.

Goal oriented planning: During the last three to four years, the executive board of the County Council has demanded that local boards formulate plans according to stated goals and objectives. A concerted effort was undertaken to do this. Goal achievement is now being evaluated and indicators to monitor and evaluate goal achievement are being developed.

Needs based budgeting: The County Council has developed a new model for budgeting, that determines resource allocation by consumption of health care services. Consumption was used as a practical approximation to health needs. The budget was based on the expected consumption of different age and sex groups of medical and psychiatric care (visits and days of inpatient care), and GP's and district nurses visits.

The model takes in account both inpatient and outpatient care. The formula had to be 'simple' in order to make it understandable. As the population size and age distribution were the dominating factors, parameters of mortality and morbidity were not calculated and were not included into the model.

The general assumption was that different PHC areas have the same expected need for health services. Thus, the county average consumption was used as a standardised value. The estimated consumption was priced and resources were then allocated to each PHC district and to different activities within the districts. Through calculating demographic changes, it was possible to use the model on a long-term basis. By putting different values into the model, for instance prices and types of standardised consumption, it was possible to direct the supply of services to, for example, more outpatient services within the health care sector.

As mentioned above, there was only one general hospital in the county. Due to long distances, there was an overconsumption from the central districts, which was taken into account. Therefore, the budget for the hospital services was set by a political decision. The character of the county and its historical development also determined the allocation of a minor part of the resources outside the model. For example, the rural districts were compensated for high transportation costs.

The new budget model was presented to the central and local boards, focusing on the policymaking elements in the formula. The model was implemented in 1992.

Monitoring: One aspect of the project has been development of quantity and quality indicators for monitoring and managerial purposes. Two types of indicators have been designed: one concerning patients opinions about

146

their visits to the PHC centre; and, the other concerning care of the elderly. Data was collected through questionnaires, one directed at patients, and the other at staff in charge of elderly care.

The first questionnaire was sent to patients one week after their visit to the PHC centre. Among other things, questions were asked about their satisfaction with the services. It was modified to include questions about whether the services helped patients to solve the problems that caused the visits and whether patients were kindly treated. The questionnaire about care of the elderly, completed by staff, included questions on decisions taken regarding social, nursing and medical support, terminal care and staff turnover.

The project was also concerned with implementing a computerised registration of all GPs and consultant visits, including number of patients, patients in need of home services and waiting discharge, as well as complications after hospital treatment.

The list of indicators developed for monitoring and managerial purposes was as follows:

*	Infant mortality rate;
*	Days of sick leave;
*	Dental health status;
*	Rate of parent support groups;
*	Rate of population having pensions before 60 years of age;
*	Rate of vaccinations;
*	Physicians (GPs and consultants)/1,000 population;
*	Rate of population where travelling exceeding 20 minutes, to GP, during working hours;
*	Amount of patients treated at each level of care;
*	Rate of patients satisfied with their visit to the PHC centre;
*	Waiting list for specified diagnoses/treatments (hip surgery, eye surgery, rupture surgery, coronary diagnostic procedures and sterilisations);
*	Complications after surgical treatment;
*	Rate of patients in hospital inpatient care waiting for discharge, needing home service;
*	Rate of re-admissions for the same problem in psychiatric care;
*	Relation between acute/planned admissions to hospital;
*	Hours used to health care planning in PHC care/1,000 pop.;
*	Cultural activities associate with the care of the elderly (nursing homes);
*	Rate of personnel/patient in home care for the elderly;

*   Rate of patients in terminal care who died at home.

Indicators have to be easy to apply in daily work. They must also be regarded as relevant by those using them. This means that all indicators must be designed in cooperation with staff. Interest to monitor one's own activities has not been great due to traditions, and lack of economic pressure or incentives. Therefore, to make indicators acceptable, the project worked with a group of representatives from different sectors of the PHC services. The group provided a supportive function regarding the implementation and acceptance of indicators by the PHC services. Implementation was done gradually, giving management and staff the opportunity to adapt the organisation to use the new information. Some of these indicators were used at the central level, to describe services in all PHC districts and in the hospital.

Conclusion

The development of a model for needs-based resource allocation took time, as it was a new way of thinking for officials and politicians, and partly overruled their power. It was important for all involved in the decision-making process to have time to discuss the effects of the new allocation philosophy. It was also advisable that politicians decided freely about the allocation of a small portion of the resources.

There was a need for clear rules about the responsibilities of the central and local levels on resource-allocation and results, as well as on what would happen if the expectations were not fulfilled. It was difficult to establish realistic goals at the central and local level; it was also difficult to define needs and measure them precisely. More work is needed in this area, but what is most important is to establish a planning model that works than to have more scientific measures.

An allocation model must take into account all resources for health care and, preferably, also resources allocated for those sectors of society that influence health, for example, social services and housing. (In Sweden, these resources are the responsibility of municipal authorities). It was difficult therefore to allocate all health care resources according to needs, as the health system is a very traditional and normative ruled organisation.

The allocation model was based on consumption of health care, as it was an easily agreed measure of needs. However, other measures that better reflect need, for example, mortality, health risks and inquiries on perceived need, should also be considered. The allocation model should be used not only at the district level, but also to allocate resources to activities within the district.

With regard to monitoring, the main conclusions of the project are: First, the building of a monitoring system should go hand in hand with the development of a needs-based allocation system, as well as with decentralisation and goal oriented management. None of these can stand alone if there is to be a successful reorientation of the organisation. Second, monitoring must take into account resource usage, performance and goal achievement at the same time, and should be part of a planning and budgeting process. Third, it is important to present to local authorities measures, figures, and comparisons between districts, early in the process, as this will help discussion and to manage organisational change.

Activities of local political boards in PHC

Kaj Norrby

Aim and methodology

The study evaluates the activity of the local health political boards. The county has decentralised political boards in the eight municipalities. Hypothetically, there could be expected a shift from budget dominated work and discussion to more strategic work and community responsiveness. This should be made possible by the decentralised situation, closer to the management of the municipality.

The local political health boards were created in 1980 to broaden the health political impact on primary health care in order to adjust the medicare system to local needs. Until then decision making in PHC was a professional, medical and administrative matter. It was expected that, in the first years, local boards would concentrate on budgeting problems, then interest would shift to organisational problems like staffing and production and lastly, activities of the local political boards would reflect more concern about local needs, local health and medicine effects community participation.

Therefore, the study evaluated the local boards work, as reflected in its protocols, in relation to the WHO targets on healthy public policy, social support systems, multisectoral policies, PHC-based system, content of PHC, and coordination of community resources. The study ran from 1981 to 1989 and all key policy documents, records of meetings, etc, were analyzed. The local boards decisions were coded as follows:

* administrative decisions;
* decision about activities in the field or health strategy;
* initiator of the decision;
* type of decision: a) positive - negative - modification or non-decision; b) administrative decision procedure or lack of procedure.

Results

The majority of decisions and discussions reported in protocols from local health boards were purely administrative, and did not deal with health strategies or activities. Only a few were strategic or about activities in the field (in 1981, 19.5%; in 1986, 20.7%; and in 1988, 27.8%). The areas of non-administrative decisions concerned primary health care activities, namely prevention activities, elderly care, and cooperation. In 1986 and 1988, decisions were positive in more than 50% of the cases. In the three years of the study, local medical doctors were the initiator in most of the decisions (Table 15).

Conclusion

The study showed that local political boards in Jamtland had difficulty in delegating away formal and administrative work, though a positive trend towards more decisions on activities can be seen. There was no evident evolution towards health promoting activities or PHC strategy, indicating a lack of local skills in community participation and cooperation. After conclusion of the study, a reorganisation of the management system was undertaken and from 1992 onwards local boards have been replaced by neighbourhood health forums.

Table 15
**Local health boards areas of non-administrative decisions, and type
and initiator of decisions**

Areas of non-administrative decisions	1981 %	1986 %	1988 %
Primary Care	21.3	11.2	8.7
Prevention	0	13.0	23.4
Elderly Care	22.0	19.2	16.3
Cooperation	2.9	12.4	1.6
Type of decision			
Positive:	30.8	51.0	50.1
Ad acta:	52.0	24.4	21.1
Initiator of the decisions			
The board itself	17.7	10.4	21.2
Local medical actors	21.2	15.1	25.4
Local lay actors	10.0	04.9	14.2

Decentralisation of primary health care

Gunilla Fahlstrom, Lennart Holmquist,
Ingrid Pincus and Anna Swift-Johanisson

Aims of the project

The experiment in decentralisation of PHC in Orebro County Council had two principal objectives: to provide a better service through greater collaborative efforts; and to enhance local democracy and local participation. Experimental projects were established in five municipalities in Orebro County. The experimental projects were evaluated over a two and a half year period by a variety of qualitative methods including questionnaires, interviews and participant observation.

Background

Orebro County is situated in the middle of Sweden. It has a population of 260,000. The County is dominated by the town of Orebro, which has a population of 120,000 inhabitants, mainly employed within service and administration. The town is divided into 15 areas each with political municipal sub-committees, with responsibility for social care, elementary schools, leisure and culture within their area. The Regional Hospital of Orebro provides all medical specialities and serves the surrounding councils as well as Orebro. There are two minor hospitals at Karlskoga and at Lindesberg. PHC is distributed via 24 clinics with at least one in each of the county's 11 municipalities.

In the early eighties the municipality of Orebro was divided into sub-districts, in order to improve the possibilities for local democracy and citizen participation. Political responsibility rests with the sub-district committee. Politicians are appointed by their party, and seats are allocated according to the results of municipal elections. The committees have responsibility for social issues, basic education, culture and leisure.

In 1986, new legislation allowed county councils to organise themselves in a similar way to the initiative undertaken by the municipality of Orebro. The County Council decided to set up an experiment with local PHC committees at Ljusnarsberg, Kumla, Brickegarden and Haga/Tysslinge. A different approach was tried at Vivalla-Lundby. Here the municipal sub-committee took over responsibility for the PHC clinic. This meant that, for the first time in Sweden, PHC ceased to be under county council control.

152

The aims of the two decentralisation experiments (Vivall-Lundby, and the four PHC districts) were similar. Both shared the expectation that collaboration between services would increase, thus providing the public with a better service and improved efficiency. The PHC committees, however, had a further objective to increase opportunities for citizens participation, and thereby stengthening local democracy along the lines of the initiative taken by the municipality of Orebro. The focal point of the experiment could thus be described as an ambition to increase the sensitivity and adaptability of services to local needs, through increased delegation and local participation.

The political committee in charge of the organisational revision had stated that the areas involved with decentralisation should differ in content and extent of work. They also stated that the experiment must take place within existing resources, and that the experiment should be seen as a 'practical investigation' (implying that solutions to local problems should be sought locally).

The first step in the implementation process was to create local work groups. These were lead by the chief medical officer and consisted of representatives from the care giving institutions involved and local union representives. After this initial stage the local work groups were meant to follow and analyse the situation, and to propose solutions for changes in the local administration and management of County Council services.

The nature of the experiment was merely political and administrative. The medical content was not changed; responsibility for these issues still rested with individual doctors. Administration and management at this level consists of: planning (staff issues, activities, research and development); budget and economical routines; and revision and control.

The PHC committees assumed their responsibilities during winter and early spring 1986. The solutions that emerged were quite different in nature from one experimental area to another.

The five districts had populations ranging from 5,000 to 18,000 inhabitants, and were anything from suburban housing areas of Orebro town to remote communities in the deep forestland of Bergslagen. In smaller areas, there were traditional PHC services (general practice, district nursing, including maternal and child health care, and some day care physiotherapy), whilst in larger areas, dental care, nursing homes and or care for the mentally handicapped were also provided.

In four of the districts, a local nursing officer provided administrative support for the board. The most radical solution was found in the largest district, Kumla, where the activities included a relatively large amount of care for mentally handicapped and a nursing home. Through budgetary reallocations, the work of the committee administrator was combined with the work of a personnel administrator, and all personnel administration for the PHC clinic and the nursing home was decentralised. A professional administrator was employed.

The experiment at Vivalla meant that PHC became a section under the municipal sub-committee. Committee administration was carried out by existing staff at the sub-district office.

Methodology

The experiment was followed by an evaluation team from the local university and the regional hospital's department of social medicine. The evaluation team's work was process orientated, following the process from the start until Autumn 1989. The evaluation of the decentralisation process in Orebro used a variety of qualitative methods but principally questionnaires, interviews and participant observation.

Seven sets of questionnaires were distributed. Two separate sets of questionnaires were issued to all committee members (N=74) and to staff (N=250) at the experimental PHC units. One set was administered at the start of the experiment, and one at the end.

A questionnaire was also sent to the union representatives at the experimental units (N=36) at the end of the project. Questionnaires were given to those involved in setting up the projects (working group members, N=40) and to a sample of the population living in the experimental areas (N=2900).

This sample was drawn from a regional population register and included all inhabitants 18 years or older that were born in three specified days of the month. The population questionnaires were sent to the repondents' home addresses, whilst all other questionnaires were sent to the respondents' work addresses.

Interviews were conducted with chairs of the PHC committee (N=5), chief medical and nursing officers (N=11), PHC committee administrators (N=5) and union representatives. The researchers also attended relevant committee meetings and educational activities, and reviewed relevant documents (conventions, regulations and minutes).

Results

The impact of the experiment was limited, but the local units have been strengthened. The majority of the population in the areas where the experiment took place were unaware of the existence of a PHC committee. Asked who they would contact if they wished to influence an issue concerned with the overall distribution of PHC, most people answered that they would contact their chief medical officer, or someone else on the staff of the clinic.

With the exception of chief medical and nursing officers, and committee administrators, few of the staff reported that they had been influenced to any major extent by the experiment. Nor had they, as reported in an initial survey, expected to be so. Staff in general had limited contacts with their committee politicians.

The local union representatives were allowed to be present at committee meetings, and most made use of this. But the overall opinion of these people was that discourse between them and the local politicians had been poor and infrequent. The evaluation showed no results that indicated any empowerment of local patient groups or local citizens' organisations.

Local politicians in three out of four PHC committees thought that their activities had been meaningful. At Brickegarden, where the experiment only concerned one relatively small clinic, politicians reported that their influence had been small, their tasks had been too few, and their responsibility had been minor. At Haga/Tysslinge the politicians also shared the opinion that the tasks had been too few, whereas at the two other areas the local politicians were rather more satisfied, believing that their work had had some impact and that the nature of their allocated responsibilities was appropriate. Both politicians and PHC staff considered that a PHC committee should be responsible for at least a PHC clinic and a nursing home.

Chief medical and nursing officers reported that the experiment had meant both increased freedom and an increased workload. Nurses who had become committee administrators reported new tasks, which meant a demand for new skills and thus further training. The medical officers in charge of the clinics of Vivalla and Ljusnarsberg were unreservedly in favour of the experiment. Others reported both negative and positive results. Increased contact with politicians was reported as an asset, whilst the time spent at meetings, and preparing for them, was not always considered valuable. All chief medical officers reported increased freedom of action.

Two of the experiment clinics have open surgeries, which allows patients to visit without having made an appointment. One of these units, on the initiative of the board, also staged an 'Open House', inviting citizens to come and talk to staff and local politicians.

Conclusion

It is difficult to determine what changes within PHC can be seen as a result of the decentralisation experiment and which changes were caused by other issues and general trends. PHC is under constant development. The evaluation covered a period of two and a half years. This is a substantial period of time, though perhaps not enough to register and analyse all effects resulting from decentralisation. It is often said that the impact of an organisational change cannot be estimated until after at least five years.

The impact of the experiment was limited, but the local units have been strengthened. Increased collaboration among political agencies did result, at least in one experimental area, but generally both staff and local politicians did not see many benefits accruing from the changes. The results indicated that local patient groups or citizens groups of any kind gained little or no improvements from the experiment.

The evaluation results also showed that PHC management had been little affected by the experiment during the first three years. Local union representatives were present at board meetings, but PHC staff knew little about the boards and also reported that communication was poor. Delegation power to local PHC management can decrease staff involvement. In certain cases the management can be an efficient hindrance allowing less information to slip down to the staff than in the earlier more centralised organisation.

An ultimate conclusion of the evaluation may be formulated thus - delegation of responsibilities to the local level provides an increased scope for efficiency and adaptability to local needs, but if a political body is to be creative there is a minimal arena below which activities are no longer feasible.

The national focus of interest among both politicians and administrators has changed since 1986, and political decentralisation has ceased to be a key issue. The experiment with PHC boards was terminated at the end of 1989. Today three PHC boards still exist, and one has been closed. The experiment with PHC under a local municipal board in Vivalla continues.

United Kingdom

Primary health care in England

The current population of England of 48 million is projected to rise to 50 million by 2001. Inhabitants over retirement age now total 7.6 million (15.5%), and again this is forecast to increase to 8.2 million (16.2%), by the end of the century. This increasing number of elderly, including those over 85 years, where a 30% increase occurred during the 1980s, presents major challenges for health care in the period to the end of the century and beyond.

Life expectancy at birth in 1989 was 73 years for males and 78 for females. Infant mortality is currently 8.4 deaths for every 1,000 live births. Immunisation uptake rates have risen steadily during the 1980s with 80% coverage for whooping couth; 85% coverage for measles; and 90% coverage for polio being achieved.

Premature deaths from vehicle accidents; cancers, in partricular breast and cervical cancers; ischaemic heart disease; and strokes are a major cause for concern. Smoking is the subject of public health promotion activitity with 32% of the population still smoking cigarettes (a reduction from the 45% in 1974). Alcohol is a major cause of ill health with 1.4 million people classified as heavy drinkers and 20% being shown to have alcohol level in access of the legal limit.

At the end of 1990 there were just under 4,000 reported cases of AIDS in England of whom 55% had died. Mental disorders constitute a major cause of morbidity accounting for 14% of reported days off work, 23% of in-patient costs and 25% of pharmaceutical costs. Obesity is increasing in both men and women with 12% of women and 8% of men being obese in 1986/87.

The National Health Service (NHS) introduced in 1948 provides

157

comprehensive health services for the entire population at no cost at the time of use and is funded largely through general taxation. Changes have occurred in the structure and organisation of the NHS with effect from April, 1991 with implementation of the National Health Service and Community Care Act (1990). Primary Care is the first point of contact with the NHS for most patients. The PHC team comprising general practitioners, nursing and professional staff provide both care and act as 'gatekeepers' for referral to secondary hospital care.

Approximately 98% of the population are registered with a GP who might be single-handed or work in a group practice with the support of the community health services. Developments in the 1980s have underlined the importance of PHC and the role of the GP in providing it. During the period from 1979-1989 there has been a 20% increase in GPs with the average number of patients on a GP list being typically 1,500 - 2,000.

PHC services are managed both by District Health Authorities (DHA) and Family Health Service Authorities (FHSA) with personal social services being the responsibility of local authorities. The population served by these three statutory organisations often do not coincide. GP services are provided by doctors under contractual arrangements with an FHSA with the contract setting targets linked to incentive payments for cervical screening, vaccination and immunisation, and health promotion. Provision of these services linked to DHA community health services highlights the need for effective working arrangements in PHC. The FHSA has a service planning responsibility which must be coordinated with that of the DHA(s) in the area covered, FHSA's frequently covering the geographical area and population of more than one DHA. In some areas where the DHA and FHSA have a common boundary, management arrangements have been closely integrated. DHAs and FHSAs are grouped into 14 Regional Health Authorities which are accountable to the Management Executive of the NHS and to the Secretary of State of the Department of Health.

Implementation of the National Health Service and Community Care Act 1990 has prepared the ground for a more strategic approach to health care. Health authorities act as 'purchasers' of health care, assessing what needs to be done to improve health, setting priorities for those improvements; and purchasing effective services to meet those needs. A typical DHA would serve a catchment population of between 200,000 - 350,000, although there are some significantly larger serving populations of up to 850,000. The 'provider' services, including hospitals, community health services and ambulance services are provided within the NHS either by management units directly accountable to a DHA or as a self govering trust. In both cases, the 'provider' has to secure contracts for its services with a 'purchaser' to remain viable.

The range of services offered by a community unit could include community-based services for the mentally ill and mentally handicapped, together with child and adult community services, including community dentistry, family planning, vaccination and innunisation, health promotion and district nursing and health visiting services.

The changes from April 1991 are accompanied by resource allocation developments, with DHAs receiving a weighted capitation-based allocation to provide services for the resident population within the area of the DHA. The DHA will therefore pay from its allocation for services provided for its residents who receive treatment outside the DHAs boundaries. GPs can also choose to be fund-holding practices through which, from the DHA allocation, the practice receives funds to purchase some hospital services.

Currently, health services expenditure account for about 13.5% of total public expenditure (5.7% of GNP and estimated to be 6.5% if private sector expenditure is included). Approximately 70% of total expenditure is on the hospital and community health services with 25% on family health services.

The Dudley Health Authority projects

The Dudley Health Authority developed two projects to 'Tipping the Balance Towards Primary Health Care', one on care of the elderly and the other on primary prevention of cardiac and arterial disease (CHD). The first project was an evalutation of the change in provision of long-term care from an institutional setting to small, locally-based nursing homes supported by PHC services, and the development of indicators for planning and monitoring the new pattern of service for this client group. The second project aimed at screening the population at risk of CHD and at promoting healthy lifestyles.

Background

Dudley, in the West Midlands conurbation of England, covers an area of 9,795 hectares and has a resident population of 300,000. Currently, 17% of the population are over retirement age and this is expected to rise to over 19% by the turn of the century with 5,000 people being over the age of 85 years. Industrial activitiy in Dudley has centred upon heavy engineering and its world renowned glassmaking, although over the last decade there has been a significant reduction in heavy engineering with associated closures and redundancies. The impact of the industrial past is reflected in the health status of the area.

Dudley comprises five townships: Sedgley/Coseley; Dudley; Brierley Hill/Kingswinford; Stourbridge; and Halesowen each with a resident population of between 50 - 80,000. The boundaries for DHA community services are co-terminous with those of the local authority, Dudley Metropolitan Borough (Dudley MBC) and Dudley Family Health Services Authority (Dudley FHSA). Joint strategies agreed by the Health Authority, FHSA and MBC have been developed since the mid 1980s, including those for mental handicap, mental health and, since 1987, elderly services. Developing locally-based services in each 'township locality' is a keystone of each strategy.

Local authority services include social care, housing education, leisure and environmental services. Health services within Dudley are provided by Dudley Health Authority (DHA) through its two management units - an Acute Service unit and the Priority Services Unit. The latter has responsibility for services provided for the elderly; mentally ill; mentally handicapped and the whole range of community health services, including health promotion. Additionally, Dudley FHSA manages the family

160

doctor, dentist and pharmacist services in the area.

Recent developments in private nursing home provision in Dudley have resulted in over 500 beds being available by mid 1990 within the Dudley boundary, the charges payable by residents in these homes being met either wholly or in part by the Government through state social security benefit funding to those residents and from payments made by the resident, or someone making payments on their behalf. The DHA accepts this responsibility for its contract beds in nursing homes.

Care of the frail elderly in community-based nursing homes supported by PHC

Jo Wood and John Daley

Background

At the beginning of 1988, long-term health care for the elderly frail within Dudley was provided on two hospital sites (Burton Road Hospital - 117 beds: and Hayley Green Hospital - 50 beds). Potential benefits for patients and a more cost effective service pattern were discussed at that time. A decision was taken to accelerate the programme for developing community-based services for elderly people by establishing a network of neighbourhood nursing homes in collaboration with the private and voluntary sectors through contractual arrangements for provision of care.

Elderly people admitted to nursing homes under these contractual arrangements were transferred from being inpatients under consultant medical care to residents in the community receiving medical care from their own GP and the PHC services. Agreement was reached between hospital consultants and GPs on the medical conditions which could be accepted into nursing home care. As a result of this shift in provision towards community care, the DHA hoped that very frail elderly people would benefit from:

* less-institutionalised surroundings;
* more privacy for themselves, their belongings and their affairs;
* more control and choice over their daily lives;
* more opportunities to do more with their lives;
* families and friends living closer to them and seeing them more frequently.

In addition, since nursing home costs were lower than those for traditional long-stay hospital wards, this shift would be a more cost-effective pattern of care, releasing funds which could be used to expand services in the community for elderly people and to provide support for carers.

In the nursing home contract emphasis was placed on the development and maintenance of a homely environment for residents with the explicit objective of securing for residents in each home the above benefits. There is a legal requirement that all nursing homes be registered by the health authority in whose area the home is located. To achieve registration, nursing homes must meet standards relating to, for example, accommodation, facilities for residents and staffing levels (which incidentally were higher standards than for inpatient care in hospital wards). The Priority Services Unit which negotiated contracts with nursing homes was not involved in the registration process and contracted only with registered homes.

Methodology

The objectives of the study were:

*   to analyse existing data about the characteristics of elderly people who had moved from hospitals in Dudley to the six nursing homes where the health authority had placed contracts at the time of the study (late 1989/90);

*   to analyse existing data about, and to observe the physical environments of the continuing care wards in the hospitals and of the nursing homes;

*   to compare key aspects of the organisational environments of the hospitals and the nursing homes which were generally considered to contribute to the quality of residential care provided for, and the quality of life experienced by, elderly people.

Aspects of the organisational environments identified in the contracts between DHA and the nursing homes included:

*   privacy for themselves, their belongings and their affairs;
*   choice, wherever possible, especially with regard to the pattern of their daily life, including times of awakening, retiring and taking meals;

*   the encouragement of regular occupational and leisure activities for
       all residents;
*   opportunities to mix with people in the community, whether by
       going out or inviting people in.

To assess key aspects of the organisational environments of the
continuing care wards and the nursing homes, personal interviews were
conducted with a total of 46 residents and 52 staff. In addition, a postal
survey and follow-up telephone interviews were conducted among 62 of
the nursing home residents' most frequent visitors; 37 (60%) responded.
A pilot study was conducted covering aspects of the hospital/nursing
home environment including accommodation; social environment
(management practices and caring routines); staff attitudes and training;
opportunities for residents to take decisions over key aspects of their
daily lives; leisure activities; access arrangements; and maintenance of
residents' skills. Information on the accommodation standards by room
sizes, availability of single rooms and toilets was obtained from each
hospital and nursing home, and compared with national and local
standards. Interviewing, using data collection instruments, was
undertaken by an external researcher.

Results

The residents: When the study commenced (September 1989), a total of
180 continuing care patients moved to contract beds in five nursing
homes. Of the 92 survivors, 39 (42%) were interviewed. During the
course of the study, a further 18 continuing care patients moved to a
sixth nursing home and seven of them were interviewed both before and
after the move. Throughout the study, a number of continuing care
patients remained in hospital and seven of them were interviewed.
   Most of the continuing care patients who had moved to the nursing
homes were women over 75. In terms of age and sex and life
experiences, the nursing home residents were broadly similar to the
continuing care patients who remained in hospital. Those who were
interviewed tended to be biased towards the younger and least physically
and mentally frail residents. In all settings, most of the surviving
residents assessed by health authority staff during the course of the study
were judged to be at the upper end of the dependency range; that is, they
were unable to do anything except wash their hands and face or feed
themselves, if their food was cut up, without help from somebody else.
   The homes: Five of the nursing homes were based in a variety of

adapted buildings accommodating between 18 and 24 people in total - only some of whom occupy contract beds. The sixth nursing home was purpose-built and accommodated a total of about 100 elderly people in living units of 30. Externally, all the nursing homes give the appearance of being more homely and less institutional than either of the hospitals with continuing care wards. The views from the lounges of all the nursing homes were also more like those from a private house than the views from the dayrooms in the continuing care wards.

All the nursing homes offer residents bedrooms rather than a bed in a large ward. Only the purpose-built home, however, offers all residents the privacy of a single bedroom. Estimates of the amount of bedroom and sitting/dining space per resident vary between the homes. In some, the amount of bedroom and sitting/dining area space per resident was greater than in the continuing care ward from which patients had moved, and in others about the same. In all the nursing homes, the furniture and furnishings in the public areas created a more homely, less institutional internal physical environment than those in the continuing care ward in hospitals.

The organisational environments

Privacy: All the nursing homes offered all residents more privacy than the continuing care wards in the hospitals to the extent that everyone had a single or shared bedroom. In other respects, the physical environments of the nursing homes appeared to offer little, if any, more privacy than the continuing care wards in the hospitals. Rules and procedures in all the nursing homes appeared to reflect as much concern for people's privacy for themselves, their belongings and their affairs as the continuing care wards in the hospitals. Some care practices noted in the nursing homes and the hospitals, however, indicated a tendency for staff concern about people's safety to override their concern for their privacy.

Choice: In all the nursing homes, waking and getting up routines appeared to be slightly more flexible and allowed residents more choice than in the hospitals. In all the homes, however, some residents' reports suggested that there was some gentle pressuring to get up at certain times. Other daily routines - for example, bedtimes, bathtimes and midday mealtimes - appeared to be much the same in all the nursing homes and the hospitals. Rules and procedures and care practices governing elderly people's freedom of choice appeared to be much the same in all the nursing homes and the hospitals, with none of the homes or the hospitals appearing to be consistently 'liberal' or 'restrictive' in the

164

amount of choice they offered to residents.

Activities: All the nursing homes made greater efforts to encourage regular occupational and leisure activities for all residents than the continuing care wards in the hospitals, but not as much effort as some residents and some visitors would have liked. There were marked differences also in the range and frequency of activities in different nursing homes. At one extreme, one nursing home employed an occupational helper four days a week to plan and organise individual and group activities during the day and evening, and over half the residents reported that they were usually involved in some daytime activity. At the other extreme, some nursing homes did not employ any specialist staff and there were no regular, planned activity programmes.

Links with the community: Visiting arrangements were similar in all the nursing homes and the continuing care wards in both hospitals, with people being allowed to visit their relatives or friends at almost any time. There was little evidence, however, that relatives and friends visited residents more frequently in the nursing homes than they did in hospitals because they had less far to travel. Opportunities for elderly people to go out were generally better in the nursing homes than in the continuing care wards in the hospitals - partly because some were situated closer to local amenities. However, the frequency with which residents were taken out by staff for local trips and for outings to more distant places varied considerably both within and between homes. While one home arranged frequent local trips for individuals and monthly group outings throughout the year, others only took residents out in the Summer for a push around the block when other duties permitted.

Overall verdicts: All the residents who stated a preference for living in a nursing home or a hospital said they preferred living in a nursing home, mainly because the surroundings were more homely and comfortable, the food was better and they had more choice. Few found anything to complain about. At the same time, many said they would prefer to live at home or in a private household. Most visitors felt that their relative or friend was as well or better cared for in the nursing home than the hospital because they had more personal attention, the food was better and there were more organised activities. Some visitors were critical, however, of certain aspects of the physical environment, the low level of activity, the lack of physiotherapy and the speed with which staff responded to residents' requests to be taken to the toilet in some homes.

Staff who had moved from hospital to a nursing home generally agreed that the physical surroundings were more homely than those in hospital and that residents had gained more privacy, more choice and more opportunities to take part in activities.

Principal indicators: The study focused upon the development of indicators relevant to assessing the success, or otherwise, of the arrangements within homes to achieve the objectives in moving to nursing home provision for the frail elderly. The resultant report was shared with the management of the nursing homes and their staff to discuss the findings and differences between homes, both to assist in raising awareness and standards and, equally importantly, to refine and agree workable indicators for day-to-day monitoring.

Costs: Comparative costs of nursing home and long-stay hospital provision indicated that the former was 70% of the cost of inpatient care. Differences in contract bed prices existed between homes, especially those where DHA employed staff were contracted to work in homes, the higher NHS pay rates being reflected in a higher cost per place than in the commercial 'for profit' homes. Market forces with the growth in nursing homes has maintained competitive rates between homes.

Accessibility: Another aspect of the project related to accessibility and it should be noted that during the study period the availability of nursing homes was confined to the western and central parts of Dudley. This restricted availability meant that nursing homes were available in only three localities and this was reflected in the study outcome. Since the completion of the study, contract arrangements have been made with two homes in eastern Dudley and a third contract became operative in mid 1991.

Conclusion

Provision of services for the continuing care of the elderly frail has transferred within Dudley from hospital consultant-led provision to a more locally-based service with residents receiving medical care from their GP and the community health services in accordance with the agreed joint strategy. Allocation of resources for the elderly frail within each 'township' locality is now being examined to ensure that needs are related to resource allocation.

Primary prevention of cardiac and arterial disease: Dudley healthy lifestyle project

Mike Smith, Margaret Marsh, J Tromans and S Ashton

Background

Screening for risk factors for heart disease has become widespread and there are a large number of initiatives in progress based sometimes on health promotion departments, sometimes on individual general practitioners practices and sometimes on groups of practices. Prior to 1987, there was no actual screening in Dudley, although some practices had well-man and/or well-woman clinics. The health promotion department in Dudley, previously had developed a 'Heart, Health and Lungs' project, (Bone, *et al*, 1988), and this had had some encouraging results with healthy motivated volunteers.

In 1987, a visit to the Oxford project impressed the Dudley team by the simplicity of their scheme to opportunistically screen individuals for CHD (Fullard, Fowler and Gray, 1987). It was decided to set up a similar project in Dudley, but to offer in addition back-up support - either by referral of at risk individuals to advisers and/or group sessions run by the Health Promotion Department. The project aims were:

* to screen the population of Dudley (age group 30-65) for risk factors for ischaemic heart and vascular disease;

* to encourage the adoption of a healthier lifestyle and thereby contribute, in the longer term, to a reduction in coronary heart disease in Dudley.

The project continues. This paper makes some attempt to interpret the outcome of the project.

Methodology

A pilot scheme was set up in an urban three-person practice in the central Dudley area. The practice had a list size of around 7100 patients and operated from two premises. The majority of the practice population were considered to be the old 'working class' (social class 3-5). Approximately 10% of the practice population were from ethnic minorities, mainly from the West Indies or the Indian subcontinent. Unemployment was high due to the demise of a large number of local manufacturing firms, in particular, those based on the iron and steel industry. This project aimed to promote healthier lifestyles by:

*   opportunistically identifying patients as they attend their GPs surgery and offering them screening for risk factors for IHD;

*   offering at-risk individuals advice on a one-to-one basis at the check-up;

*   offering referral of at-risk individuals to advisers and/or groups (dietician, stop-smoking) for further or ongoing advice;

*   appropriate medical advice or treatment for previously undetected medical disorders.

After the initial contact with the Blekinge team, which carried out a similar project, it was decided to include routine screening for raised serum cholesterol in the study. Resources in Dudley (as everywhere in the United Kingdom) were very limited. It was confirmed with the local biochemistry department that random total cholesterol was the simplest and probably the best indicator to measure and that the cost was low. The researchers were uncertain as to the long-term value and/or safety of lipid-lowering drugs and therefore did not plan to treat high cholesterol with drugs but rather to see the effect of dietary advice. A nurse facilitator commenced work in December 1988. The facilitator's role was to ensure effective coordination between groups and the health promotion department, and to provide the training and support to practice nurses. Additionally, the nurse facilitator had responsibility for the establishment of procedures and practices of the screening programme. In March 1989, the facilitator sent out a questionnaire which revealed a few practices to be offering well-person clinics but with little attempt being made to fully screen their populations.

The health promotion team developed the back-up support programme in collaboration with the GPs and the practice nurse. A community dietitian independent from the rest of the team, agreed to give dietary advice to those with very high serum cholesterols, or those with complex problems.

Results

At the outset of the study in September 1987 there were approximately 3000 patients in the age group 30-65. All those attending were offered advice and information regarding diet, exercise, smoking cesation and alcohol consumption, as appropriate. The team also found previously undetected hypertension, diabetes, raised blood cholesterol, familial hypercholesterolaemia, and initiated the appropriate action(s). Early follow-up of those with raised serum cholesterol level has been successful, in most cases. Whether this initial achievement will be maintained over the years remains to be evaluated.

While patients were reasonably keen to attend one-to-one sessions with the practice nurse, they were considerably less enthusiastic about attending group educative sessions or other advisers. The dietician has been of considerable value but people rarely seek referral for smoking, exercise, stress or a combination of these. Therefore, the response to other sessions organised was very poor and over the latter part of the study no further attempts were made to continue them.

The role of the Health Promotion Department (HPD): As a result of a previous project on the prevention of CHD, the staff of the HPD had gained experience in working with the community on an educational approach to lifestyle and the socio-economic factors which influence health behaviours. It had shown that well informed, well motivated people already know the key health messages. What they had identified were practical difficulties which prevented them from acting on health messages that they already agreed with in the first place.

The team was anxious to see if this experience could be helpful to the GPs screening programme. The work was based on the self-empowerment model - helping people who volunteered to attend regular self-help groups; to acquire new knowledge and skills which would enable them to make beneficial changes. Following screening, the GP and the practice nurse gave patients verbal and written information and advice, and referred or recommended individuals to attend 'self-help groups'; for example, to receive help in giving up smoking. Many individuals said they would like to give up smoking but found it difficult to do so on their own. Some needed ongoing support for weeks/months, before they succeeded.

The HPD set up self-help groups, led by a health professional. Group sessions were designed to exchange ideas and learn from each other, with support from health professionals, to find answers to many of the difficulties people were facing. Often it was a case of stimulating motivation and self esteem and highlighting the benefits to be obtained from a healthier lifestyle, but it was also recognised that there were many socioeconomic factors outside the control of the health service which made it difficult for individuals to adopt health messages.

The group sessions worked on the basis of making small changes, gradually over a period of time and were non-threatening. Unfortunately, after an initially enthusiastic response from a small group of women, the group sessions failed to attract sufficient numbers of participants to make them worthwhile. Attempts were made to modify the format, and leaflets advertising the sessions were circulated, but this brought no significant response and the sessions were abandoned. More success was achieved in advising patients individually at their initial screening session with their GP.

Discussion

The Oxford project (Fullard, *et al*, 1987) has shown the benefit of screening the general public and offering health education advice as appropriate. The Dudley project cannot be fully assessed as completion, at time of writing, was at least one year away. That this project was someway behind on its target is due to the absence of the practice nurse for several months: the wish to keep waiting lists for screening appointments short. In a practice where pressures on reception staff were great and surgery lists inevitably long, it was not always easy to be motivated to spend time explaining the rationale behind the screening programme. Recognising the time limitations of the GP and practice nurse, the health education contribution was to provide an opportunity for patients to exercise and discuss ways of improving their lifestyles.

The following are some of the difficulties and reasons why the group sessions offered were poorly attended. Whereas in the previous Health, Heart and Lungs project, group sessions proved very successful with well motivated, well educated people in employment and a reasonable income; the area targeted this time contained a high proportion of lower socioeconomic groupings, some living in, or experiencing, difficult and distressing conditions. It was very difficult to attract those individuals to attend group activities because health does not feature strongly in participants needs until they become ill. They rely greatly on the doctor for their health and do not recognise that they can make a contribution to their own health in partnership with their doctor. Some people who perceived themselves to be 'healthy' (as in the absence of illness) thought health education should be for people with health problems. They had a medical model perception of health and did not appear to value the contribution they could make by working in partnership with their doctor to prevent or reduce the risk of illness or disease. They did not see group sessions or educational activities as part of their culture.

Men were particularly reluctant to take part in group sessions. They had preconceived ideas about exercise sessions and were more likely to want to exercise alone. Compared with some of their daily problems, patients saw the potential dangers of smoking, for example, as unimportant and in fact they saw smoking as helping them to cope. Low incomes did not enable the participants to have much choice in food and in some cases basic cooking and preparation skills were poor. This is a reflection of the socioeconomic factors already mentioned in the practice area.

Some patients saw health professionals who ran group sessions, as presenting a middle class image, or as 'busy bodies' who could not relate to their real needs. The team tried to identify one or two members of their own community who might train to work with their own people - but with little success.

Conclusion

Opportunistic screening of CHD is beneficial to patients. In what concerns the development of community self-help groups, using existing community based networks appears to be a useful vehicle for getting health messages across. These are likely to be in tune with community needs, not professionally defined needs. Health on its own does not appeal to many members of the community. Perhaps linking enjoyable entertainment activities with the health message would make them more attractive and less threatening. Information-only activities have limited value, people need more than knowledge - they need to develop skills and require ongoing support from health professionals. Simple, practical approaches are more likely to be effective. Goals must not be set too high; if they are difficult to achieve they destroy motivation. If possible, activities should be on a neighbourhood basis and easily accessible.

A fundamental approach to the project was to do more than an information giving exercise exercise, and to attempt to provide opportunities for patient to participate more in acquiring new skills for the management of their own health. General practitioners did not have the time to give this level of on-going support.

The experiences of the project have led to further development of health promotion initiatives in the community, and have influenced: first a local project starting in 1992 to maximize individual, family and community

171

potential for health, and to develop coordinated PHC/school/community networks which can provide long-term locally based lifestyle education programmes; and second, as part of a national GP led PHC initiative, which involves providing PHC workers in planning team activities in prevention and promotion, stimulating inter-professional teamworking; and managing available resources.

The North Staffordshire Health Authority (NSHA) contributed with three projects to 'Tipping the Balance Towards Primary Health Care'. The first was about decentralisation of PHC, and sought to: assess the appropriateness of introducing locality management in community health services; and, canvass the perceptions of managers and staff on the benefits derived. The second project introduced neighbourhood forums in order to reorientate health service decision making to more fully reflect the needs of the community. The third project was one of several initiatives in North Staffordshire aimed at reducing a perinatal mortality rate which was around double the national average for the United Kingdom. Its focus was provision of common health messages and support for behaviour change in women of childbearing years.

Background

The NHSA is one of three health districts in the County of Staffordshire. Within its boundaries are three district councils, the City of Stoke-on-Trent, the Borough of Newcastle-under-Lyme and Staffordshire Moorlands District Council. Each of these Local Authorities serve communities which have distinct social, industrial and geographical profiles. These contrasts are also reflected in the comparative health status of the population.

The City of Stoke-on-Trent comprises six quite distinct towns whose historical and present day industrial base is in the production of ceramics. The City and its environs are known as 'The Potteries'. Coal mining is another major industry, and there has been a history of migration to service the labour demands of the mines and factories. In recent years economic recession has taken its toll, although it is now in a period of recovery, with the creation of new light industries. The city has large municipal housing estates on its periphery which exhibit high levels of social deprivation.

The borough of Newcastle-under-Lyme comprises a large market centre and residential area together with a small town and scattered villages. It is virtually a continuation of the City, much of its population are engaged in pottery and mining industry. The Staffordshire Moorlands District Council has three main population centres of between 10,000 and 25,000 population. It has a sparse and declining population, who are largely dependent on agriculture and its attendant industries. Within the

Moorlands is some of the United Kingdom's most beautiful upland countryside, which is used for leisure purposes.

The NSHA embraces an area of 88,000 hectares, and nearly 470,000 people, making it the largest district in the West Midland Regional Health Authority, and the sixth largest in the country. The NSHA has six units of management consisting of two acute units, mental health, mental handicap, elderly care and community health units.

The NSHA in collaboration with the City Council has recently completed a health profile of the population of Stoke-on-Trent. Similar projects are being carried out in Newcastle and the Moorlands. The Stoke-on-Trent study, combined with other epidemiological data shows both significant health problems and inequality in the life experience of the population. The City has an overall standard mortality rate (SMR) some 25-30% above the comparable national rate. Within the City there is not an electoral ward that enjoys a level of health better than the national average. Some wards experience SMRs 40 to 50% higher than the national average. The situation is better in both Newcastle and the Moorlands, though areas of quite high deprivation exist in both.

Decentralised locality management in community health services

Amanda Kemp

Background

The aim of a decentralised approach was to provide community health services that were efficient, effective and responsive to local health needs. The 1980s have witnessed a myriad of national influences which have lead community health services to examine the relevance of decentralisation - or locality management - to meet the challenges facing the NHS. The national influences were:

* criticism of bureaucracy in the NHS. Smaller decentralised management areas would be able to be more responsive to the local market place;
* the drive to contain costs within the NHS;
* the acceptance by all political parties of the need for innovation and responsiveness at local level;
* the publication of the Griffiths Report in 1984 emphasising the need for health services responsive to local need;

*   the ever increasing wish by local people to be involved in the
        community

Three recognised features of decentralisation have been used by general
managers in the NHS as tools to provide effective, efficient and
responsive to community health services: the localisation of service
delivery; a lower level of management within the organisation; the
structuring of organisational relationships to possibly include generic
management, working and budgeting. In addition, the involvement of
people of all disciplines and at all levels in the NSHA organisation was
required so that they felt free and able to question the way services were
provided.
    Locality management in North Staffordshire was designed to be the key
to a decentralised structure which would be responsible and effective to
the needs of the population. The 460,000 resident population of North
Staffordshire was divided into three localities to provide community
services. Each locality has a locality general manager.
    Locality general managers were given responsibility for: local budgetary
control; control over staff establishments; the responsibility to develop
proactive links with other statutory and voluntary agencies; the ability to
review and restyle services as appropriate to local need. Therefore, the
locality general manager position was one with the power to deliver local
health services appropriate to the needs of local communities.
    A further important theme in the particular decentralisation model
adopted was that of democratisation and the involvement of the local
community in services via the introduction of neighbourhood forums. A
structure of local management within a community health service setting
might appear to be a panacea for combating the diagnosed ills of public
sector bureaucracies. However, the selection of the method of
decentralisation was only the first step on the ladder of introducing a
decentralised management structure. The difficult task was its
implementation and sustained operation. How the structure actually
functions and the impact it has must be evaluated in order to ascertain if
the original objectives were being met.

Methodology

The evaluation research on the decentralisation structure focused on two
important aspects. First was an assessment of the appropriateness of
introducing locality management into PHC services. This organisational
review draw upon techniques used in strategic planning to examine both

the external and internal environment to see whether decentralisation was the 'best fit' organisational structure for community health services.

The second area of investigation focused upon the perceptions of managers and staff within the organisation as to whether decentralisation and its themes of delivering management power and associated features has actually occurred.

The assessment techniques that were used included structured interviews of all managers with the organisation. A postal questionnaire survey was also distributed to 760 staff. The questionnaire was a national survey which was made available to the National Health Service in 1990 by the Department of Health.

The questionnaire was designed to find the attitudes of people working in the organisation. It built upon an organisational review questionnaire which had been used in private industry with alterations to meet the specific needs of the NHS. Seven key areas of people's attitudes were measured: goal alignment; good communications; initiative; teamwork and trust; adult treatment; personal development; service reputation. These key themes and their scores are indicators of how well an organisation is functioning in each of the areas. Clearly, the higher the score, the more effective staff perceive their organisation to be.

A response rate of 74% was achieved. Results of the survey were available for each management area and staff grouping, broken down by age and length of service. An enormous amount of data was therefore available to be used within the organisation.

The first measurement of perception was undertaken in July 1989. Two further evaluations involving all management and staff were carried out in October 1990 as a major component of a project funded by the Department of Health. The outcome of the introduction of decentralisation and its overall acceptance by management are discussed in the sections that follow.

The move to a decentralised structure

Any change in organisational structure needs to take account not only of relevant external national issues but also the local factors that are apparent. Only by reviewing the influences at work at different levels in the NHS will the organisational structure be obtained which 'best fits' the environment prevalent within the organisation and give it its best possible opportunity of achieving its desired aims. One of the strengths of decentralisation is that it can be adopted and adapted in a form which is most appropriate for its environment, both within and without the organisation.

In moving from a centralised to a decentralised structure, the organisation goes through the realms of design, culture, climate, development and strategic planning. It is also evident that in moving through these phases the organisation should be in a continual process of learning, reviewing, adapting and readapting to the environment.

Audit of organisational performance

It is not easy to evaluate organisational performance. However, it is important to establish an evaluation framework since this can offer new management strategies and could lead to further enhancement of the functioning of the organisation. In North Staffordshire, an initial evaluation of the attitudes of managers was carried out. Work elsewhere (Carnall 1990) bears out the relevance of evaluating people's attitudes towards the organisation in assessing the review of organisational structure and functioning.

The HAY organisational climate questionnaire, used to evaluate and improve the adequacy of PHC in Kuwait, has been used as an initial basis for evaluation. The main thrust of the HAY approach is to measure the perception of what people actually feel is happening within an organistion. Therefore, an organisational climate review should confirm whether or not the key elements of the role of the local general manager are perceived by people working in the organisation. The HAY model was incorporated with an evaluation framework or audit put forward by Elcock (1988). The audit tests staff perceptions and attitudes on two main areas:

*   has local management moved decision making from a centralised to a decentralised base?

*   does decentralisation give the opportunity to truly develop services that are responsive and appropriate to local communities?

The audit was distributed to 27 managers within the unit. The managers were all the senior and middle managers in the organization. An overall response rate of 88% was achieved with 24 completed audits returned. The responses to the audit indicated that there was considerable commitment to decentralisation from all the groups within the unit.

Table 16
Responses to the organisational audit

Statement	Agreed or Strongly Agreed
Managers are encouraged to innovate	95%
Decision making is innovative	75%
Managers are willing to experiment with different ways of providing services	70%
I feel as though I work in an innovative organisation	79%
Locality management has allowed decisions to be taken at a lower level	75%
Locality managers are accountable for the services of the Locality	83%
It is important for localities to continue to have control of resources to allow services to be developed which are responsive to local circumstances	91%
Decentralized management has produced unquantifiable benefits of:	
* local decision making	77%
* participative management style	77%
* increased control of resources	77%
Locality management has the delegated power to respond directly to the problems encountered	77%
Locality Management has developed a strong base in the Unit	65%
A decentralized structure gives the Unit the best possible opportunity to develop local links with other agencies	78%
A decentralized structure gives the Unit the best possible opportunity to provide services responsive to the needs of local communities	83%

Decentralisation was perceived as being something tangible rather than management rhetoric (Table 16).

In North Staffordshire, community health services locality management appears to be achieving the main objectives of decentralisation. The unit is innovative, gives individuals responsibility and, most importantly, has shifted decision making to a local 'generic' manager who has the ability to provide services that are responsive to the needs of local communities.

The audit responses confirm that decentralisation can work if the organisation is truly concerned to make itself more responsive and is willing to introduce an organisational structure that alters the nature and manner of the services it delivers.

It is important that the organisation accepts the relevance of regularly assessing whether it is functioning in a way that enables it to achieve its objectives. Therefore in October 1990 further evaluation work was undertaken within the unit. Structured interviews were undertaken with both the 27 managers who were involved in the previous research and a further 13 managers within the unit. A 100% response rate was achieved. The structured interview covered peoples opinions towards four key areas:

* acceptance and understanding of the organisation's management arrangements;

* the communication methods that were used by the interviewees within the organisation and their effectiveness;

* the identification and the relevance of the objectives of the unit;

* the accountability for service delivery in the organisation.

Analysis of the interviews confirmed the results that were previously achieved. The key themes that emerged from the interviews were:

* continued strong commitment to decentralization;
* a clear understanding of the levels of accountability and who takes decisions in service delivery;
* a high level of delegation and responsibility;
* an organisation that obtains results by communicating with people to achieve action rather than relying upon written communication;
* an open and participative style of management;
* locality management has developed and enhanced relationships with

179

external organisations (such as social services, voluntary organisations) that are essential to community health services.

Thus the themes of decentralisation were still both meaningful and functioning within the unit. The open and participative style of management, a fundamental aspect of decentralisation, certainly was in operation. Decentralisation facilitated and enhanced key elements of the 'healthy' organisation; such as achievement, clear accountability, a management structure that was appropriate to the task, and good communication. The survey also highlighted relevant issues at which management needed to work, if it is to continue to function effectively.

In October 1990 a communications survey was carried out among all staff within the unit. The aims of the survey were to develop an understanding of attitudes and opinions towards the functioning of the organisation. A response rate of 70.8% was achieved from the 760 staff who were asked to participate in the survey. Table 17 describes the seven main areas of measurement of attitudes and perceptions and the benefits that positive scores in these areas make towards an effective organisation.

The staff communications survey highlighted certain strengths and weaknesses with the move to decentralisation, especially at the lower end of the organisation hierarchy (Table 18).

The information indicates that only 34% of people responding to the survey knew the goals of the unit; 52% felt that communications were good; and 59% considered that the unit actively fosters personal development. The four scores over 55% record a very positive attitude towards the organisation. The management style of decentralisation and the issues that it is tackling had a direct impact upon the way staff view the organisation and their personal development.

The results at North Staffordshire Community Health were very high scores compared to the national results that were returned from the units who participated in the survey throughout the country. The high scores were not just returned from managers in the organisation. From the analysis of the data, it could be seen that similar scores were returned from most staff groups. The similarity of scoring is indicative of the principles of decentralised management which have been adopted throughout the organisation.

Table 17
Perspectives of decentralisation

	Ideal State	Benefits
Goal alignment	Everybody in the Unit pulling in the same direction: Individual, professional, unit and section goals relate to the unit's mission and strategic vision;	Builds cohesion, efficiency and effectiveness of all activities: Provides direction for planning and individual efforts;
Good communications	Clear, sufficient and appropriate information flows top-down, bottom up and laterally throughout the unit;	Necessary requirement for success - basic to establish and maintain an appropriate unit culture; A common theme running through all factors;
	All communications are read and watched and understood;	Can move the needle through all other factors
Initiative	Opportunity and 'permission' to think for themselves and help the unit address problems in areas where they can make a difference;	Provides opportunities for for innovation and self-esteem; Increases the Unit capacity to adapt and respond under changed circumstances;
Teamwork & trust	People talk and work together in functional and multi-functional groups with cooperation and honesty;	Builds sense of 'comfort' among staff; Improves organisational efficiency and effectiveness;

Adult treatment	Each member of staff is treated with dignity and respect;	Prevents feelings of anger and frustration that cause withdrawal of commitment;
	Controls and rules make initiative, sense;	Encourages teamwork, pride and confidence.
Personal development	The Unit provides staff with the opportunity to develop new/current skills;	Prepares people to be more effective; Builds optimism about the future and enhances commitment;
	The Unit encourages staff to develop themselves within and outside the day to day organisational environment;	Economic benefit;
Service reputation	All staff possess a sense of kinship with patients and a real understanding of their needs. They understand the Unit's services and their work is perceived as ultimately driven by patient needs;	Creates staff who are more likeley to feel loyal and committed; Gives them sense of their own worth; Delivers better quality patient care;
Emotional profile	Emotional state under which staff operate;	Enriches understanding of the seven factors;
Morale index	Indicates how staff feel about morale in their immediate working environment.	Useful summation of the climate.

Table 18
Staff communications survey

Objective	Perceptions of achievement (%)		
	Positive (>55%)	Weak (40-55%)	Negative (<40%)
Goal alignment			34
Good communications		52	
Teamwork & trust	59		
Personal development	66		
Service reputation	77		

183

Conclusion

The money spent on the payment of salaries in the NHS represents nearly 79% of the total expenditures. It is therefore essential that people working in the organisation feel positive towards its objectives and the philosophy of management.

The work on management structures in North Staffordshire has shown that staff feel positive towards the outcomes that are being produced by the structure. Table 17 has clearly defined the benefits of achieving positive scores. These scores are achieved equally in all managerial and staff groups. The positive scores served to reinforce the results of the organisational climate audit that had been carried out the previous year. Together the results indicate that all the key features of a well functioning organisation are working in North Staffordshire.

It is important that the organisation continues with an annual review of the perceptions of the people working within the unit and to act upon the issues highlighted by it. Only by being prepared to review its capabilities will it be able to deliver the best possible health care to its population.

Increasing local democracy through the introduction of neighbourhood forums

Marjorie Gott and Glenn Warren

Aim of the project

Health care delivery in the United Kingdom has been criticised as being both too patriarchal (professionals decide what people want) and not really health care, but illness care. In terms of budgeting and policy making, preventive (community health) services are afforded scant attention, as opposed to (hospital based) treatment and curative services. In addition to the relatively low status and funding of community health services, there is currently a growing debate about their purpose. This debate is underpinned by changing notions of the meaning of health and health work, and changes in the role and relationships of health workers, both with each other and with clients. What we are seeing is the 'unfreezing' stage of a social change phenomena, as community health workers seek to interpret and respond to the principles of the Ottawa Charter. This is the contextual backcloth against which the Neighbourhood Forum Local Demography initiative was developed. Its aims were as follows:

* to give members of the community the opportunity to influence local public service health decision making;
* to reorientate local health service decision making to more fully meet the expressed needs of the community;
* to increase partnership in local health related planning, service delivery and review.

On their own, the forums were seen by the unit to be of little significance if not matched by supporting intra and inter-organisational changes (Baric, 1990). Some of the necessary support changes were the focus of other TTB projects. Briefly, the areas of internal organisational change which were seen to allow the growth of activity around the forums were:

* Decentralisation of the management structure with the creation of local 'general' managers;
* Decentralisation of budgetary control - over 90% of all budgets are now managed by local managers;

* Development of an 'open management' style - it was seen to be essential within the organisation if 'openness' was expected at Forum level;
* An integrated management development programme - to empower managers at local level;
* Development of effective information systems covering both activity, health and social status, both available to allow for local area/neighbourhood analysis;
* A strong emphasis on boundary management.

On an intra-organisational level, the areas of activity have included:

* Local managers strengthening ties with voluntary and 'not for profit' organisations, both in terms of time and financially;
* The support and funding of community development activities;
* Positively identifying areas of joint activity with other agencies, including:

> joint funding of health and social profiles; joint newsletter for community health staff, social service, GPs, dentists, pharmacists, opticians, housing, environmental health and voluntary organisations; reviewing joint planning structures to

ensure that they emphasised 'partnership'; joint campaigns; development of a radio 'soap' which highlights social and health issues; and the identification of joint use premises.

Methodology

The difficulty of getting representative local participation was recognised at the outset and the strategy chosen was to identify, through a multiplicity of contacts, existing networks. This proved to be very successful in identifying a wide and diverse range of contacts, with groups from adolescents, through to the elderly being represented. One of the most useful contacts proved to be the Council for Voluntary Services, who provided a rich range of networks.

In addition to trawling people through known networks and personally inviting them to attend a Forum meeting, the date and time of meetings, together with an invitation for anyone interested to attend, was widely advertised in frequently used public places such as, post offices. In this way it was hoped to attract members of the community who were not directly in receipt of a health related service, but who might, in any event, want to participate in decision making about their local health care.

The instruments chosen to measure degree of, and views of participation in, local decision making were: checklist to be used during actual meetings by a non-participant observer; and a interview schedule to be used for individual face to face interviews with participants.

The checklist was an existing instrument developed to measure the degree of participation in, and effectiveness of, meetings between school staff, governors and other interested parties making decisions about education (Williams, 1984). The interview schedule was developed for the purpose of this study, piloted with a small number of people, then redrafted. Sample size was 49 interviews (an approximate one in four sample from six of the now 14 forums) and 15 observations of Forum meetings. Both types of data were drawn from all six Forums in the study.

Results

Both direct observation data and data collected by personal interview show that Neighbourhood Forums were successfully achieving their aims of increasing local involvement and partnership in health related decision making, and of addressing those needs which communities themselves had identified. As stated above, a random sample of attenders (49) was selected for interview. The characteristics of this group were as follows: the majority were female (32) and in the 40-65 age group (30). There were few people over retirement age (5). Attenders were mostly professionals (health service 13, other public sector 23). Of the health service professionals the majority were nurses. Public sector representation included teachers (5). Ten members of the community were interviewed, including three local councillors.

Interview data: The preponderance of professionals was sometimes remarked upon adversely by people when interviewed. It should be noted, however, that some Forums were just beginning and, as they had been initially instigated by the Community Health Unit staff presence was necessary to support group cohesion, development and, ultimately, self-management. It is also worth noting that there was very strong representation from other professional groups. This was highly valued and seen as the origins of an extensive public sector network that could make public services more efficient and effective in identifying and responding to community needs.

The believed purpose of the Forum was seen as improved service coordination (26), improved communication (17), to meet community needs (18) and to enable the community to help itself (12). Responses (substantiated by Checklist data) indicated that the purpose of the Forums was clearly understood. The believed membership was seen as predominantly professional (49). In answer to the question; 'What kind of people come to these forums?' a Home Help responded; 'Mostly the High Ups, except for me and a helper from Sheltered Accommodation'.

Her view was echoed by a lady who worked as a cleaner in the community: 'A lot seem to be educated people with responsible jobs like health service workers, community (government) workers, head teachers, police, and social workers. Myself and other people like me come, but sometimes we find it is a bit above us ...... however you do need people in authority as they can get things done'.

Also mentioned as attending meetings were voluntary sector workers (19) local councillors (16), lay people (14) and clergy (14). Others who should attend were seen as local residents (26). In particular young people (6), young marrieds (3) and the elderly (1) were mentioned. Other suggestions included local shopkeepers/chemists/ publicans (7), police (6), local industries (3) and family doctors (3). Some people, when asked, stated that no-one else need come, the community was well represented. Below is a typical response:

Whilst we are interested in the service of the individual client in the community, if each meeting included all members of the public then there is the risk that the forum would degenerate into a talking shop for individual complaints, whereas, in my view, the Forum is to act as a sounding board of local opinion to feed back to the health authority views about the health service and to make suggestions for improvements (clergyman).

Community participation in decision making was seen as occurring by 16 respondents. A further 14 felt that there was potential for it to occur, but Forums were only just developing. When asked why they had responded in this way, two main sources of substantiation were offered. Sixteen cited new services that had developed as a direct result of the setting up of the Forums, and 10 offered the opinion that, as a result of the Forums, local resources were being managed better: 'A local handicapped group needing premises has discovered facilities available in a local school at a favourable cost, of which they were previously unaware ... improved communication brought the need and the facility together' (teacher).

'Mothers attending the Health Centre complained that their pushchairs parked outside were being stolen. A system has now evolved of marking the pushchairs and of locking them. This was pioneered by the Police Crime Prevention member of the Forum and is now likely to be used elsewhere' (clergyman).

A few people (three) believed that although the Forum did allow the community a say in health related local matters, some of the issues raised were beyond their power to deal with, as they required investment in the structural quality of the environment. The need for adequate street lighting to reduce the incidence of both accidents and crime was identified. A local councillor made a general comment about the power of the group to effect change. 'I have a positive feeling about the meeting but ... their success depends on a lot of things.... I think the Forums need a higher profile with the support of the right people with the power to get things done'.

Whilst it is true that the Forums were only consultative bodies and do not have either a budget, or a mandate to change statutory public service provision, it was clear that, for a lot of members, they were working by both making better use of resources available and by finding creative and flexible ways to change services. They have also had some success in attracting funds: 'There is always the frustration of fund raising, but this Forum has just been awarded £500.00 by the Prince's Trust' (observer).

Questions on defining health and health services were included to identify what concepts of health attenders held, how closely these matched the aims of the Forum (reorientation), or traditional health services (care and cure). It is interesting that attenders generally had broad conceptions of what they meant by 'health', thought the Forums shared this broad understanding, but defined the health service in the neighbourhood almost exclusively as members of the PHC team (community doctors and nurses). These findings indicate that the Forums were successfully reorientating attitudes towards and within the statutory community health services, but that some designated health carers, in particular PHC workers employed and managed by general practices, may remain marginalised in relation to this new area of work and of thinking.

Definitions of health centred on wholeness and wellbeing in mind, body and spirit (26), and being able to function/cope (30). Three people spoke of complete fitness and absence of disease, whilst the view of 13 was much broader and more in line with HFA philosophy. They said - all aspects of living in the environment (10), and the welfare of the whole community (3): 'Health is related to all aspects of life and living ... to live in a good community with support when you need it .... to be able to be happy and contented in oneself, contentment both physical and mental. It involves good housing, sufficient income and appropriate support' (housing association official).

Views on Forum attendance were positive with over half the people interviewed (30) saying that they had learned as a result of attending. Of this group most (20) spoke of learning about extra resources available to improve the health of the community, and of learning more about different workers roles and functions. Ten stated that they now realised that the community was very diverse and they appreciated other peoples problems more. Seven remarked that there was a lot of previously untapped motivation and goodwill to draw on.

Networking was quoted as a particularly useful function, half of those interviewed saying that they had made new contacts as a result of attending meetings, and a further six saying that they valued the opportunity to meet contacts face to face. Views on the Forum as an intervention were positive: from the 21 taking up the opportunity to add unsolicited comments at the end of the interview, 17 were positive (ranging from good to brilliant idea!); 'Forums are an excellent way forward to meet the needs of the community. We must listen to the public to see how we can help. Forums will help us do this I give them full marks' (police officer): 'I think the forum is a tremendous idea. All credit should be given to the health service for starting and launching it.

The locality manager has given it a brilliant start' (youth worker).

Observation data were collected by non participant observers who attended meetings and used a checklist to record observed behaviours. The checklist comprised 25 items plus space for additional comments. Items were grouped to give the following categories: common purpose; common agreement; shared commitment; active participation; group cohesiveness; leadership/management/efficiency (business matters).

A four point Likert scale was used, ranging through strongly agree to strongly disagree. Responses were heavily predominant in the two agreement columns, with strong agreement being accorded to three of the eight active participation items: mutual interest was shown in all members points of view; the atmosphere was supportive and helpful; members were interested in the meeting. There was also strong agreement observed in what concerns the shared objectives of the meeting, and shared commitment to those objectives. The following comments (taken from different Forums) are typical:

> 'Seventeen people attended and all participated in the discussion. Discussion was animated and there was a measure of agreement on the issues which were important. However many held back from taking concrete action and the chair had to work hard to get a subgroup appointed to carry matters forward';

> 'The group appears to have gelled well. Members work together in a constructive and business-like atmosphere';

> 'Very well organised group. Although some members offer more in the way of input to the meetings there was a feeling that these people are expressing sentiments mirrored by others within the group therefore maintaining cohesiveness';

> 'This was a very positive and supportive meeting ... there were definite members who took a more active part in the discussion'.

The above comments are indicative of cohesiveness and common purpose. Some also indicate the importance of good leadership and management skills. With two exceptions, all meeting observers reported good group leadership and management. Qualities noted included focusing on issues and the use of creativity and flexibility in arriving at solutions. The exceptions were Forums where the chair was felt to be too inflexible and autocratic.

The observer said; 'The meeting, I felt, caused frustration. The format made no allowance for questions A presentation on the role of the nurse and the role of the health visitor took up most of the time, and the time factor blocked any questions'. The observer correctly identified none of the participation criteria as having occurred at this meeting. In another meeting, the observer identified strong leadership as evident, but perceived the chair as pursuing his own agenda; 'Street traffic became an issue in the B area for 15-20 minutes because, I think, the chair person is on the Council Highways Committee'. As noted, however, these views were in the minority. Most comments noted the facilitative abilities of the chair.

Conclusion

The findings indicate that the North Staffordshire Neighbourhood Forum project was successful in its initiative to increase local democracy in health related decision making. Whilst some problems had been identified the indications were that as these Forums evolve, problems will be tackled by the broad coalition of members.

The principal problem was the need to increase the attendance and involvement of local residents in the neighbourhoods. The difficulty of reaching 'the community' has been well documented (Wynn Williams 1988). Forum members were very mindful of this and designed a number of strategies to improve the attendance of local people. These included the delivery of a household information sheet and questionnaire, a newsletter, and a personal invitation to parents to be taken home by local schoolchildren. The community unit now provides substantial financial support to the three councils for voluntary services to underpin these interventions.

Community participation is not easy to measure as attendance at meetings is only one criteria. Bichmann *et al* (1989), working in collaboration with WHO and UNICEF, are developing ways to measure community participation. They identify key features as needs assessment; leadership; organisation; and resource mobilisation and management. Many of the detailed criteria for successful participation that they identify have been noted in this paper. The implications of the findings are that both the intervention (Neighbourhood Forums) and the research design have wider applicability for successful implementation in other communities within and outside of Britain.

191

Reducing perinatal mortality - a community initiative

Alison Norman

Aims of the Project

The project aimed to effect a further reduction in perinatal mortality within North Staffordshire Health Authority by promoting pre-conceptual care in the community. The specific objectives of the project were: to agree the content and range of health messages to be used in relation to pre-conception care; to improve the knowledge base of PHC professionals with regard to the pre-conception care messages and the need for consistency; to develop, with PHC professionals, methods to promote on an opportunistic basis, the discussion of pre-conceptual care with potential mothers and ways to help them introduce the messages into their particular lifestyles; and to increase the number of women who plan for their next pregnancy by adopting the pre-conception care messages. Although the project focussed on perinatal mortality, the general approach was to encourage a healthy lifestyle, thereby impacting on other areas not necessarily specific to pregnancy.

Background

In the past two decades perinatal mortality has reduced in the United Kingdom. However, in comparison with other developed nations the rate remains high; and the perinatal mortality rate is higher amongst social classes 4 and 5 than social classes 1 and 2. It has also been noted that there is considerable variability between mortality rates from area to area, This phenomena is well illustrated by North Staffordshire (Table 19). The 1988 rates for both the Region (West Midlands) and the District are significantly higher than the national norm. When the North Staffordshire District is further divided this variability is even greater; 1989 shows a marked improvement, but a better comparison is probably provided by the 1987-1989 period average. It is also important to note that in 1988, 27% of births in North Staffordshire were to single women.

Factors associated with perinatal mortality may be both clinical and socio-economic. These include access to health care, availability of neonatal intensive care facilities together with lifestyle issues, such as smoking, nutrition, economic status and social support. Whether or not the pregnancy is planned, together with the age of the mother may be crucial. The interrelationship of these factors is complex but most

Table 19

Perinatal mortality in North Staffordshire

Perinatal mortality	1988	1989	1987-1989
England & Wales	8.7	8.3	8.7
West Midlands Region	10.3	9.7	10.0
North Staffordshire	12.1	9.7	-
Borough of Newcastle-			
under-Lyme	7.9	10.0	10.2
City of Stoke on Trent	15.8	9.7	12.0
Staffordshire Moorlands	5.9	8.4	9.1

Compiled from: OPCS Tables, Vital Statistics for West Midlands Regional Health Authority, North Staffordshire Residents, 1987-1989.

authorities now agree that socio-economic factors have considerable impact on the likely outcome of pregnancy. For example, Whitehead in 'The Health Divide' (1988), refers to indicators such as high unemployment and poor housing as being closely associated with high perinatal mortality rates. Similarly, the West Midlands Regional Health Authority Regional Report on perinatal and infant mortality (1983) cited deprived social background as an indicator of possible low birth weight and increased perinatal mortality. Furthermore, an analysis of the population of North Staffordshire, using the Jarman 8 Index Score (1983) highlighted a high correlation between low, birth weight and socioeconomic deprivation.

The Regional Health Authority Report highlighted the need to reduce smoking, improve the amount of exercise taken and to influence the nutritional standards of parents in order to try to combat high perinatal mortality rates. A further issue that is linked to high perinatal mortality both by the West Midlands Regional Health Authority and the National Third Report of the Social Services Committee (1984) on perinatal and neonatal mortality is that the pregnancy should be planned.

Therefore, the promotion of pre-conceptual care and the adoption of a healthy lifestyle seems to be a relevant prerequisite to continuing a healthy pregnancy with a resulting higher birth weight child. A further issue to promote is to encourage people to use the family planning services offered by general practices or community services. Furthermore, we thought that all the professionals involved in providing antenatal care should have the same level of knowledge and information to give to parents on lifestyle issues such as smoking, alcohol, exercise and diet.

The intervention

In designing the intervention the strategy was as follows: to set up a multi-professional working group to oversee the development and implementation of the strategy; to devise and implement a pilot survey to ascertain knowledge levels amongst professionals and members of the public followed by seminars to discuss pre-conception care messages and how best to disseminate them; to evaluate the survey and seminar and based on the outcome of this, run further such events in other areas of North Staffordshire.

The multi-professional working group: Membership was drawn from GPs, paediatrics, midwifery, community services, health education, and the community health council. The group has overseen the developments ensuing from the seminars. Various other activities have been generated by the group such as improved nutrition leaflets for staff/clients, a health handout to all school leavers, and activities around the promotion of family planning, (for example, making facilities more user friendly and encouraging uptake of services by younger people). All of the activities carried out were linked in order to encourage people to adopt a healthy lifestyle, which should influence the likelihood of reducing low birth weight.

Pilot survey: The survey was carried out in areas of deprivation: Fegg Hayes and Knutton/Cross Heath. In Fegg Haynes, the 22 members of nursing staff from the health visiting, midwifery, district nursing and school nursing teams attached to the health centre were surveyed. In Knutton/Cross Heath, questionnaires were completed by the 13 community nurses who work in this area. The questionnaire examined knowledge on clinical and lifestyle issues related to antenatal care. The clinical questions are used in examinations by both the Royal College of General Practitioners and the Royal College of Gynaecologists and Obstetricians to award the maternal care qualification to general practitioners. The questionnaire was felt to be very difficult and too clinical in its orientation.

Overall, the Fegg Hayes results indicated an adequate level of knowledge on clinical and lifestyle issues. The level of knowledge was excellent in what concerns the use of nicotine and alcohol both prior and during pregnancy. All respondents knew that smoking is associated with low birth weight babies, and over 50% of the respondents correctly noted nicotine and alcohol as the two most commonly used drugs both prior and during pregnancy. The level of knowledge was also high on nutritional issues. All respondents identified at least one food item which would increase dietary intake of iron, calcium and vitamin C. There was good basic knowledge about physical exercise. However, there was the misconception amongst professionals that exercise must take place on a daily basis. Some gaps were identified in knowledge related to recent advances in gynacology and obstetrics, particularly in the application of recently developed imaging techniques and therapeutics. Therefore, it would be relevant to consider study days to update community health professionals in both clinical and lifestyle issues related to prenatal care.

In the Knutton/Cross Health area, the overall results reflected very similar scores to those recorded in the first survey. The mean score for the clinical section of the questionnaire was 44.5%, and the mean score for the lifestyle section was 59.6%. A high level of knowledge was found in questions related to infant feeding and to immunization.

Seminars: The first part of the three seminars that followed was used to feed back the survey results, to highlight areas where knowledge seemed deficient and to congratulate staff where their scores were higher. The rest of the seminar comprised input from a dietitian (nutritionalist), a medical practitioner with experience of working in areas of high deprivation, and a health educator. An information pack was also distributed. This included items on nutrition, vegetarianism, smoking, use of alcohol and drugs during pregnancy and benefits of exercise.

In the first seminar, the group work proved very valuable in addressing lifestyle issues as pertaining to the local community. Key points drawn out included the belief that health services professionals, working in isolation, would not be able to impact on the lifestyle factors affecting perinatal mortality. Staff found the input beneficial but no specific strategies were implemented following the seminar.

At the second seminar, membership comprised the same as the first seminar with the addition of midwives and GPs. The following proposals were put forward as being a appropriate response to the problem of perinatal mortality in Knutton: establish a multi-agency approach; reach members of the public through a health and fitness campaign; develop parenting skills through education at schools and pre-conceptual care; action on reduction of smoking; raise awareness about the importance of pre-conceptual/ante-natal care by employers; and carry out a locally based survey on lifestyle.

A further seminar took place in April 1991. The emphasis of this was on the prevention of unplanned/unwanted pregnancy.

The consumer questionnaire: Parents attending the Infant Welfare Clinics in the Knutton/Cross Heath area, were asked to complete a questionnaire that tested knowledge of alcohol, nutrition and exercise. Some 58 parents completed the questionnaire. The answers showed a high level of knowledge regarding good health behaviour. However, this knowledge is not necessarily translated into actual behaviour. Over 90% of the respondents recognised the importance of reducing alcohol intake both prior and during pregnancy to increase the possibility of having a healthy child. Over 70% of the respondents knew that this is advisable to cut down on the consumption of fat, salt, and red meat, and that it is advisable to eat fibre, fresh fruit, salads and vegetables. About 40% of the respondents smoked. One of them stopped smoking completely during pregnancy, eight managed to reduce their level of smoking, and 13 continued to smoke at the same level during pregnancy as they had done previously.

The exercise initiative: It was agreed that health service staff participate in exercise with members of the local community and offer support for a healthier lifestyle.

Development of parenting skills: The second seminar indentified problems with the community's knowledge and expertise in the areas of nutrition, hygiene and home safety. A meeting was held with representatives from the Education and Social Services Departments to confirm to the areas of concern outlined at the seminar. It was decided that the best means of addressing the issue was to achieve a broad constituency of support, both in terms of the identification of problems and the means available to address them.

Therefore a Neighbourhood Forum was started and one of its first actions was to set up a multi-agency group to examine the problem in depth. The group initiated 'drop in' sessions, which included information on lifestyle issues influencing low birth weight.

Reduction in smoking: Arrangements were made in collaboration with a local school to involve children in a smoking initiative which includes role play. Workshop participants felt that work in schools to prevent children taking up the habit would be more productive than attempting remedial action with adults.

Raise awareness of the importance of pre-conceptual/ante-natal care by Employers: An approach has been made to a large factory whose largely female workforce assembles wires and cables. In May 1990, 39 women, currently working, were pregnant and 48 were on maternity leave. In August 1990, 53 women were expecting children. From February 1991 a programme of ante-natal care, support and advice was offered, on site, every four weeks. Despite intensive work by the midwives, the programme stopped after nine months. Even though care was provided at the factory, women did not attend because they were more concerned about the high level of redundancies occuring at the factory at that time.

Conclusion

The perinatal project had a number of successes. A multi-disciplinary working group was formed. Seminars took place and various collaborative initiatives were implemented. Work continues. A major task for the future will be the need to find means of measuring changes in behaviour patterns. Perinatal mortality rates will be monitored, but it is recognised that there may be some variation, which cannot necessarily be attributed to lifestyle change.

High rates of perinatal mortality are influenced by many causes and this intervention alone is not likely to reduce rates but should be seen as one of a number of interventions which are necessary. Adoption of healthy lifestyle habits can be influenced by personal choice and, therefore, a general improvement in health status may be expected. However, not withstanding this point, the impact of low income and other economic and environmental factors on the ability of people to modify lifestyle, cannot be underestimated.

West Lambeth Health Authority projects

The West Lambeth Health Authority contributed two projects to 'Tipping The Balance Towards Primary Health Care', both in the area of community participation and skills for PHC. The first paper describes a 'bottom up' initiative aimed at provision of community responsive PHC following sampling of local 'lay' opinion. In the second project, a short stay/local day care centre was provided to extend current PHC services. The aim was to keep people who were in need of professional health care in the community and to provide a locally based medical/nursing service.

Background

West Lambeth Health Authority (WLHA) has a population of approximately 167,000. It covers the western half of the London Borough of Lambeth and runs from Waterloo in the north to Brixton in the centre, Clapham in the west and Streatham in the south. Lambeth is an inner city borough with all the characteristics normally associated with an inner city; namely, poor housing, high unemployment and a low-level of owner-occupied accommodation. The central and northern parts of the district have been designated an area of inner city deprivation by the Department of Environment. In 1983, Lambeth ranked as the fourth most deprived local authority in the country.

Lambeth has one of the highest proportion of one-parent families in the country; 32.4% of all households compared with the national figure of 14%. Just over four percent of the adult population are on the Council Handicapped Register. Evidence shows that social deprivation and stress in inner city areas are associated with poor health (Townsend, *et al*, 1982; Whitehead, 1988). The standardised mortality rate shows Lambeth as having one of the highest rates in London. Among the 192 health authorities in the country, Lambeth ranked 32nd in the infant mortality and 58th in the perinatal mortality rate. In 1987, the perinatal mortality rate was the second highest in London.

The Greater London House Condition Survey (1979) showed that about 12,000 dwellings in Lambeth were unfit, over 12,000 were in need of major improvements; and, 8,000 were lacking basic amenities. Lambeth has a very high level of homelessness. Seventy two percent of those housed in temporary accommodation were single parent families and four perdent were single and vulnerable (physically or mentally handicapped); twenty four percent were two parent families; and fifty percent of single homeless households consisted of black people.

The WLHA covers only half of the Borough of Lambeth. Services related to health including environmental health, social services and housing are provided by the London Borough of Lambeth. Family doctor services are provided by a Family Health Services Authority which also provides support for dentistry, pharmacy and optical services. Acute hospital services are now broadly based on St Thomas' Hospital, community services are managed within and from the South Western Hospital and adult mental health services are managed within and from Tooting Bec Hospital.

The patch project: an exercise in lay decision making

Rosemary Dun

The aims of the project

The Primary Action Towards Community Health (PATCH) project was a two-year pilot scheme based in Clapham. Set up in 1985, its main task was to look at whether decentralising community/PHC services to smaller geographical areas or patches would make them more responsive to local need and facilitate collaboration between different agencies and professional groups. Patch-based health systems in 'Third World' countries have often produced startling improvements in public health (WHO, 1988). What they have in common are decentralised health systems, locally recruited community development workers, and locally elected health committees making local health decisions. PATCH wanted to find out what, if any, lessons could be learned and applied to inner city health care systems in London.

Missing from any debate or action was input from the general public, consumers, and from PHC workers. It was felt that decentralisation strategies, boundaries, and priorities were being imposed from the top down onto local communities with little analysis of whether this was appropriate. What might 'bottom-up' perspectives look like and would grassroots priorities match those being decided for local communities and people? A concern was that the vital role state health services play in promoting and attaining good health for its populations had slipped in prominence in the rush to streamline services.

The PATCH project decided to seek local opinion on health and what affects health in the neighbourhood of Clapham and to then examine the implications for health planners and policy makers. The guiding

200

philosophy for the project and subsequent health survey was the WHO Health For All definitions with their focus on community participation and intersectoral collaboration, the need to redress inequalities in health, and the importance of environmental and socio-economic factors as determinants of health.

When deciding research priorities and identifying sample populations, the PATCH project drew on local community development work. Background work revealed that terms such as 'community', 'PHC', 'health' and 'health needs' meant different things to different people and professional groups. Little was known about lay definitions. What might they be, and would they match or mismatch those of professionals? The defining of these terms became a starting point for the research. Professionals and lay people were invited to offer their own definitions and views.

Measurements of intersectoral collaboration were sought by asking workers their opinions on the way in which they worked together as professionals and across agency boundaries. Suggestions were invited for ways of improving work practices. Consumer and professional satisfaction with existing local health services were measured, and the view points of people with disabilities and their carers were particularly were noted.

The PATCH project assumed that equity in provision and representation was a prerequisite for redressing inequalities in health. Studies in the United Kingdom (Townsend *et al* 1982; Whitehead, 1987) have linked material and social deprivation with ill-health and found that discrimination according to social groupings can determine whether statutory health services are received; in particular, a study by Dun, (1984) found that middle class people are more likely to receive NHS services than those who are working class. Therefore, public opinion according to social class, disability, age, sex, occupational status, race, and housing tenure was obtained in a sample representative of the distribution of these groups throughout Clapham. This enabled analysis of any differences or similarities between socio-economic sub-cultures. Were health priorities different between social classes, age groups, sex and others? What might the implications be for NHS planners and managers whose priorities are dominated by a medical culture that was white, middle class and male?

The project was able to gain access to voluntary sector networks as a community heath initiative. But, in attempting to straddle the NHS, social services and the voluntary sector, the project failed to fully gain access to any. There was no clear commitment to implement any of its findings.

The more obvious constraints and limitations were those of time, lack of perceived status, and resources. Lack of status made access to information held in the public health department difficult, and led to problems in gaining the cooperation of GPs and other NHS staff.

Methodology

Research was carried out between October 1985 and May 1987, along with the rest of the PATCH project development work. A full account of the procedures used in the project can be found in 'Pictures of Health' (Dun, 1989). From summer 1986 to February 1987, focus group were arranged with local residents, health and social care professionals and community groups, to establish the relevant issues to be covered in a local survey, and to identify the survey populations.

Five survey populations were identified: the local population of Clapham Town and Larkhall electoral wards, (approximately 25,000); health workers at Clapham Manor Health Centre (N=50); workers at Area 4 Social Services office (N=30); local community groups from the grant-aided voluntary sector [these were selected in order to reach under-represented groups such as black and ethnic minorities, lesbian and gay communities, people with disabilities, young people, elderly]; and, key informants [people who are identified as having useful and pertinent information: community leaders, police, school teachers, primary care workers, clergy and others] (N=30).

The general trend in this type of research is to focus on quantitative data (Curtis, 1983, Betts, 1985). The survey, in an attempt to avoid limiting people's responses, used open-ended qualitative questions to elicit perceptions on health. Core questions were asked in the five questionnaires in order to allow comparisons to be made. These questions included: What is meant by health? What affects health? What is meant by community? What are local health problems? What solutions might there be to local health problems? Do local people have enough say in the health services they receive? Would they like more say? Do PHC workers have enough say? Should health and social services work together? Should statutory and voluntary sectors work together? Should PHC workers and citizens work together? What do local people and PHC workers think of the local health services that they receive? Professionals were asked about collaboration at local levels, and were also asked to suggest ways of improving working practices.

From June to September 1987, data were collected from the five populations. A research and opinion poll centre was commissioned to carry out the household survey of a representative sample of the local population, by face-to-face interviews. The local population sample was selected from the electoral register, based on age, sex, country of origin, and housing tenure. The sample size was $N=277$, which approximately represented 1:100 of the general population. The questionnaires were conducted by post, and were addressed to all members of the other four survey populations previously identified (health workers, social services workers, local community groups, and key informants).

Data analysis was carried out from August 1987 to February 1988. Data from the household survey were analyzed according to age, sex, class, occupational status, disability, career status, ethnicity, housing tenure and colour. All this enabled data analysis according to social and socioeconomic groupings. Further analysis of the qualitative data from the household survey and the questionnaires completed by the other four groups were clustered, to allow comparison between the responses of the residents and the responses of the professional and community groups purporting to represent community interests. From the responses, categories were produced, allowing quatitative measurements to be deduced. From a random sample of 50 household questionnaires, and from the professional response, it was possible to construct coding frames for the unstructured questions. There was enough uniformity in these qualitative responses to do so. In most cases the first three responses were taken.

Results

Definitions and perceptions: Lay and professional viewpoints were radically different. In some instances they were reversed. Lay people offered broad definitions of health. Time and again they referred to environmental and socio-economic factors as affecting their health. Concerns of housing, low income, pollution, unemployment, came at the top of their priorities - often above those of diet, exercise and smoking. When priorities were grouped, lay people gave environmental factors top rating. On the other hand, professionals emphasized services and lifestyle factors. They gave environmental ones bottom rating.

Professionals often felt frustrated and powerless by their perceived inability to alleviate health problems rooted in socio-economic and environmental causes. The improvement of personal and public health is beyond the scope of the NHS alone. Health professionals, managers and planners should work with others in housing, state benefits, environmental health, debt advisers, social services, police and voluntary and community groups. Partnerships between sectors and between service providers and consumers at local and central levels were seen to be crucial. As was the involvement of lay people at all planning stages.

Lay people and PHC workers largely felt that there was such a thing as geographically defined local community. They differed on the question of size. Local people identified areas of 1 to 3 streets, or their housing estate, or their route to the local shops or pub and back. Service community boundaries were 10,000 to 25,000 population whereas service user 'community' size was nearer 1,000 to 2,000 or less. Clearly boundaries need to be smaller - patch based or grouping of patches - if the aim of decentralisation is to involve local communities and respond to local need. Communities need to be involved in the drawing up of geographical service boundaries.

The population: Population groupings were examined according to class, race, sex. disability, carers, age, marital status, housing tenure, occupational status. The findings supported other research and suggested that inequalities in health persist. Inequalities in provision and representation were also likely if typically under-represented groups were not reached - such as homeless and rootless, black and ethnic minorities, single parents, children, old people, young people, people with disabilities, gay and lesbian communities. Health managers and planners need to update their information on their population splits and community development strategies to reach these populations. Robust equal opportunities that go beyond sex and race were important.

People with disabilities and carers: Working class people were twice as likely to be disabled and nearly three times as likely to be informal carers. Most informal carers were working class, women, and married; a high proportion were black. Working class people with disabilities experienced more poverty, were likely to be more ill, and were most likely to need community support services. But, in the sample group, not one person with a disability nor a single carer was identified as receiving any community health services. And, two thirds receive no additional help at all - not even from family, friends or neighbours. Chronically sick and disabled people experienced most dissatisfaction with the services they receive. People with disabilities were three times more likely than the rest of the population to think that their GP service was poor; carers were twice as likely to think so. Informal carers were four times more likely to feel that other health services were poor.

Levels of satisfaction: The general public were mainly satisfied with their GPs. They were more likely to express dissatisfaction with other community health services. The reverse was expressed by professionals.

204

They mostly felt that district community health workers did a better job than GPs. These health workers also thought that local GP service was poor.

Collaboration at primary care levels: A general feeling was that health professionals were difficult to engage with. In Clapham, PHC workers expressed a lack of 'team spirit'. But social service workers did feel part of a team. There was dissatisfaction with working relationships between health/social services and between statutory/voluntary sectors. Reported gaps and duplications in service added to an overall picture of poor collaboration. There was virtually no joint planning or working with local authority housing and environmental health officers, and little awareness of any need for this. Health and social services workers put forward their own solutions and training needs. These included coterminous boundaries, regular, formal and informal meetings, inclusion in each other's induction schemes. Increased collaboration was generally regarded as a 'good thing'.

Accountability and participation: The general public felt that they did not have enough say in local services; they wanted more. Professionals in health and social services, and voluntary sectors workers felt the same. An overwhelming majority of PHC workers felt that they should work together with local people and communities to set local health priorities. In Clapham, primary care workers from health, social services and the voluntary sector, all supported the setting up of a local public health alliance/forum, based on community health worker posts and project, to promote action. Such a project to be accountable to the local community and would attempt community involvement and collaboration at local levels. 'Pictures of Health'? (Dun, 1989) goes some way towards suggesting developments in structures, strategies and processes.

Pitfalls: The major pitfall of the project and research was that there was no commitment to follow up the findings. It lacked status and remained on the margins of NHS planning and policy. Through its development work the project was able to gain some access to district planning by being on the steering group for a Lambeth-wide Health Profile through researching and publishing a report on community work (Dun, 1987), and by attending and taking part in local national and international conferences. Papers were written and regular progress reports presented to the Health Authority.

Gaining the active participation of local communities requires time. The PATCH project was limited to two years. There was not enough time to fully involve local communities, so the health survey was not fully owned by those communities. If it had been, they could have used the findings

205

as they felt appropriate. Community participation should empower local populations. Health surveys that fully involve communities can have a strong role to play. The PATCH project tried to avoid this pitfall by involving local groups and three Clapham-based forums.

Conclusion

The project and research clearly demonstrated that lay and professional viewpoints differ. Without lay viewpoints, services and priorities will be based on assumptions and professional opinion, a result being that many needs will remain unrecognised and unmet, with any improvement of services benefiting only those already in receipt of services or well able to access them.

Inequalities in health and inequity in provision are likely to prevail without a commitment to redress the balance. Communities are not homogeneous and health services and planning need to reflect their diversity. Health authorities need to know the population they serve, and to target under-represented groups.

According to public opinion, socio-economic and environmental factors were as important to health as personal ones. The NHS cannot hope to tackle these issues alone. Collaboration and partnerships between agencies, sectors, the public and professionals all are needed at local and central levels.

Even though most people want more say in the services they receive, their level of involvement will vary. Community development strategies must reflect this. Communities are not out there waiting to be involved. Many are busy just surviving. It is important to take time over community development and participation if heath authorities are to avoid exercises that only involve listening to the same groups and seeing the same faces. Communities and citizens need to be empowered to engage with state services. Many find tackling medical staff and large institutions too daunting. Many do not try. Often a state service like the NHS can be inaccessible because of cultural, class or language barriers. Community development and community health workers play a vital part in empowering and improving access.

Community participation runs from market research type surveys, holding public meetings, involving community groups, setting up local accountability structures, through to full decentralisation of health services through the electoral process. What is important is that public opinion and community involvement is obtained at all levels of health planning and policy making. This does not, of course, mean interference in clinical or management decisions but partnerships to find joint solutions to jointly agreed health priorities. What is required is a commitment from health authorities to full community participation, to community development strategies and to setting up the necessary structures to enable public opinion to inform decision making. Hand in hand with community participation should go a policy to get contracts with client based targets, quality assurance and consumer satisfaction measurements. What is required is a change in thinking so that a climate is created whereby opportunities to involve communities and consumers are made and seized.

Primary and community care workers have a wealth of local knowledge and information. On the whole they have little or no access to health policy decisions affecting their locality and work. Their potential community development skills remain under-developed due to clinical workload and lack of status attached to community development work. Structures need to be set up to enable them to be involved in local health planning and to enlarge their community development skills. This will also involve collaborative working with other professionals and agencies.

Accountability structures are very important. Locality planning groups and/or community health forums need some real power and control if they are to avoid being a 'rubber stamping' group or 'talking shop'. This could involve something like the management of a local community budget. Structures need to be in place for locality planning teams/community health forums to input and have access to more centralised health planning.

A general plan of action for health authorities that emerged from the study can be summarized as follows:

* that health authorities adopt a stated philosophy to include a commitment to community participation, to intersectoral collaboration, to address inequalities in health, inequalities in provision and inequalities in representation;

* that lay involvement is at every level of health planning, including drawing up boundaries; deciding health priorities; identifying need; and deciding what information is collected and how;

* that health organization decentralises and responds to smaller geographical areas;

*   that accountability - over and above financial accountability - is developed at all levels of planning and service delivery;

*   that a community development approach is adopted by health authorities. This will include an overall community development strategy; the encouragement of community health workers posts;

*   that robust equal opportunities policies are adopted that go beyond sex and race to include class, disability, sexuality, colour and religion, and that will seek out views from under-represented groups, in particular people with disabilities - whatever their age or type of disability - and their carers.

Tipping the balance from central to local, from medical to health models, from professional to lay, from hospital to community/PHC, from inequalities to equity, from discharge to care in the community, are all necessary to promote health. The involvement and empowerment of local communities and consumers is essential for this to be achieved.

An assessment of community participation in an inner city PHC facility

Gregor Henderson and Maryrose Tarpey

Aims of the project

In October 1988, a 18 month evaluative study of the Lambeth Community Care Centre began. The evaluation set out to identify and assess the extent to which the Centre was achieving its main aims, and then make recommendations to help the Centre to better achieve its aims (Henderson and Tarpey, 1990). This paper assesses the extent to which community participation in the life of the Lambeth Community Care Centre was achieved and what steps were deemed necessary to help improve community participation. A number of valuable lessons can be learned from illuminating the Lambeth experience in relation to the role of community participation in attempting to shift the balance of resource provision from the secondary health care sector to the PHC sector.

Background

The Lambeth Community Care Centre opened in July 1985, and was developed as a new type of PHC facility. It was planned as a place that would treat and care for people whose illness or condition did not need acute specialty based care, like that provided in a local district general hospital, and for people who were not able to live on their own or be cared for in their own homes by their relatives, friends or neighbours without help.

The Centre was seen as an extension of a person's home where people using its services, and their carers, were involved in the planning and management of their care, and where staff worked together in the assessment, treatment and care of people referred to; it is a local community resource. Local people were encouraged to use the Centre for their own activities and enabled to take an active part in the daily life, planning and decision making processes of the Centre.

The Centre formed one part of the community health services provided by the WLHA. The Centre served a population of just over 80,000 people, and consisted of 20 inpatient beds, 22 day care places and a range of outpatient and day unit departments, namely; occupational therapy, physiotherapy, dental, speech therapy, chiropody and social work. The areas surrounding the Centre showed higher than the national average figures for adult unemployment, overcrowded homes, elderly people living alone, ethnic minority communities, semi-skilled and unskilled workers and one parent families. In terms of mortality indices, the Centre's area was higher than national average figures for deaths from injuries, suicides, cancers and respiratory diseases, with coronary heart disease being the most significant cause of premature death.

The Centre was managed by a management team (CMT) which consists of the senior nurse, one GP representative, a community/lay representative, a therapy staff representative and the Centre administrator. All referrals to the Centre's inpatient, day care and outpatient physiotherapy and occupational therapy services took place through one of the 39 GPs or 9 GP trainees who had signed a 'contract' with the health authority. The contract gave the GP referring rights to the Centre and covers the GPs role vis-a-vis the Centre and their duty to retain at all times medical responsibility for the patients they refer.

From December 1985 to April 1989 community participation was facilitated by a full time community linkworker, whose role was to link the Centre with the community and the community with the Centre (Nixon, 1986). The establishment of the post of community linkworker was an acknowledgement that in relation to health and the provision of health care services, local people were more often than not excluded from the planning and decision making process. This exclusion was due to social relations and processes, and to the development of a state of dependency on those who provided health care services by those who used them.

The community linkworker's work set up a formal structure through which people from the local community became actively involved in the planning and decision making process of the Centre. A Centre Advisory Group (CAG) made up of local people, Centre users and representatives from local community groups was established, with the express aim of enabling local people to have a formal structure through which they can influence the planning and decision making of the Centre. This group of people met on a regular basis with Centre management and put forward local people's concerns and needs.

Members of CAG were elected for a period of three years and there were seven community seats, three for representatives of local community or residents'/tenants' groups and four seats for local residents, ex-patients, patients or carers. Three staff members were also elected to sit on CAG. Each of the four professional members of the Centre's management team automatically become a member of CAG and were expected to attend the monthly CAG meetings to answer questions and to listen to CAG's requests.

Methodology

The evaluative study chose a pluralistic approach as the most appropriate method of evaluation (Smith and Cautley, 1985). This approach recognises that there were a number of differing views and perspectives on what the aims of the Centre were and the extent to which the Centre was achieving its aims. In order to take account of these differing views a wide range of people were involved in the evaluation process.

A detailed account of the methodology is given in 'Assessing the Lambeth Community Care Centre' (Henderson & Tarpey, 1990). Over the 18 months evaluation period, 41 individual and nine group interviews were carried with a wide variety of people who were using, working in, managing, or affected in some way by the existence of the Centre. They comprised three groups or 'clusters' of people: Centre users (inpatients, day patients, outpatients, relatives, carers, and Centre group users); community groups (CAG members, local CHC representative, community linkworker, representatives of group meetings in the Centre, and representatives of local community and voluntary groups); and service providers and managers. These groups were formed of three sub-clusters; primary care team (GPs, GP trainees, and FPC respresentative, and district nurses); local authority (local authority councillors and social

210

service staff); and health authority (health authority members, managers of priority services unit, hospital consultant medical staff, representatives from Centre nursing, therapy and administrative staff, and members of the CMT).

Once these three clusters of groups of individuals were identified, a sample of 41 interviews was agreed, ten of Centre users, ten of representatives from community groups and twenty one of service providers and managers.

The interviews were carried out by two researchers following set instructions and a detailed topic schedule.

The 41 individual interviews were semi-structured and tape recorded, lasting on average 40-60 minutes. The interviews were transcribed, checked against the recordings and systematically analysed for content by indexing each of the interviews by person and subject.

The nine group interviews were made up of between four and six people. Each group was constructed for the study and consisted of either a group of Centre users, Centre staff, GPs using the Centre or managers. The interviews were taped and systematically summarised, but not fully transcribed. The group interviews were analysed by content similar to the method used for the individual interviews.

A variety of other methods were used to supplement and inform the data obtained from the individual and group interviews. These included: reviewing background papers and relevant documents and minutes of meetings, carrying out systematic observations of meetings, case conferences; and, the day to day work and activities of the Centre. Both researchers were based in the Centre and therefore had a detailed first hand insight into its 'culture'. Observations were made of the major processes taking place, who the key players were and most importantly what the outcomes were with regard to community participation.

Community participation was felt to be dependent on ensuring that the Centre's services were accessible to and appropriate for all sections of the local population and that there were effective formal and informal mechanisms in place that enabled the local community to take an active part in the planning and decision making processes of the Centre.

Results

Community participation in the Centre: The involvement of the local community, voluntary and community groups and statutory organizations, was a vitally important factor in the development of the Lambeth Community Care Centre. Some of the people interviewed recalled that

211

one of the original pressures to build the Centre grew initially from an articulation of local people's feelings following the closure of the local Lambeth Hospital in 1977, that some kind of local health care facility was needed to serve the needs of local residents. The local Community Health Council (CHC), a statutory body responsible for representing local people's and patients' views, along with a number of committed local GPs, tenants groups, community and voluntary agencies, trade unions and local people campaigned vigorously for nearly 10 years for a local PHC facility.

The development of the Centre and its stated objectives reflected this 'grass roots' community action initiative, and to the Centre's credit, the identification of the aim of community participation in the evaluative study three years after the Centre was opened illustrates the extent to which the continued involvement of the local community in the life of the Centre was considered to be an important element of the Centre's life and work.

In the evaluative study, community participation was felt to be one of the main means by which local people could be encouraged and enabled to reduce the influence of health care providers and increase the influence of those who use the services and those who live in the local area. There was a general feeling in the study, especially amongst the community representatives interviewed, that active community participation was easier to achieve in a local PHC setting (like the Centre) than in a more formalised acute hospital setting.

Resources available to achieve community participation: Whilst the participation by the local community in the life of the Centre was considered to be a major aim, on close examination, the allocation of resources to achieve community participation belied this claim. Two examples illustrate this. First, the community linkworker's post was funded for three years through the Department of Environment's Inner City Partnership Scheme. When the funding for the post ended in 1989, the WLHA decided that they did not have the resources to continue funding of the post. Second, the work of the CAG was not supported by any financial assistance, even though the CAG was considered to be the main structure through which community involvement in the Centre was assessed. Each year the CAG votes on which one of its members will sit on the CMT. Although the CMT meets weekly for three hours, no travelling or loss of earnings or other expenses were made available to the CAG representatives who sat on the CMT.

A number of community representatives interviewed felt that if community participation was to be achieved, then there was a requirement to resource some of the mechanisms by which active community participation can be achieved. By providing resources, three important benefits emerge. First, it underlines a level of commitment by those responsible for providing and resourcing the services that community participation is a desirable objective; second, it illustrates a willingness to share financial responsibility with representatives of the local community; and, third, by resourcing initiatives aimed at achieving community participation, credibility with the local community can be established by those who allocate health care resources.

Access to the Centre: In both the individual and key group interviews it was felt that to bring about active community participation, local people had to have access to and knowledge of the Centre and its services. The first problem, in terms of access to the Centre, arose from trying to identify which community the Centre actually served. Those people who were on the patient list of a GP contracted to the Centre could be considered to be one 'community'. However, this excluded those people who lived in close proximity to the Centre but who were not registered with a contracted GP. To solve this problem, all local GPs in a defined geographical area were encouraged to become attached to the centre. This met with limited success, with eight GP practices within a 1.5 km radius still not contracted to the Centre. The number of patients on these non contracted GP practice list is just over 33,000. This compares to a total list size of nearly 50,000 for contracted GP practices within a 1.5 km radius.

The main reason for GPs not entering into a contractual arrangement with the Centre was the requirement that they provide 24 hour medical cover to their patients in the Centre. District nurses interviewed in the study cited numerous cases of people changing their GP so that they could have access to the Centre. This practice, whilst actively discouraged by local GPs, was encouraged by the district nurses. At the time of the evaluative, it was very difficult for someone to change to another GP. New legislation currently in place enables people to change GPs more easily. In Lambeth, this is likely to result in more people choosing to move GPs so that they can, if they need to, be referred to the Centre.

An alternative solution discussed in the study interviews was for other PHC workers (for example; district nurses, health visitors; home helps and social workers) to have referral rights to the Centre. Centre staff were ambivalent about such a policy and the majority of contracted GPs were opposed to the idea. Centre staff and GPs were concerned that such an open referral policy could lead to an unsustainable increase in

213

referrals.

A second problem identified in the study which impeded access to the Centre was the perception amongst some of the community representatives interviewed, that the Centre was a facility for the 'disabled elderly'. In the first set of interviews this was seen as a deterrent to other groups of people who might use the Centre or become involved with it. GPs felt that this perception was based on hearsay. However, there was concern amongst Centre staff and GPs that this perception of the Centre could become a self fulfilling prophecy. This view was felt by some of the community representatives and carers interviewed to be disconcertingly 'ageist' in tone. They felt that the Centre was most successful in providing care to the local dependent elderly population, and in relation to 'intermediate' care provided in a PHC facility that this was the population most likely to be using the Centre's services.

Alongside the debate on who had access to the Centre ran a parallel discussion in the interviews on the 'ethnocentrism' of the Centre's services. The 1981 Census data shows that in the Centre's immediate geographical area, 18% of the heads of households were born outside the United Kingdom. Local authority estimates were that 30% of the local population was Black. The Centre was seen to be offering services based on the needs of the white elderly population. Little attempt was made by the Centre to reflect the multi-cultural and multi-racial nature of the local community. In view of this finding the CAG decided that more positive action should be taken to redress this imbalance. However, as yet, no significant changes have been instituted.

Information: In both the individual and key group interviews it was repeatedly stated that community participation was only possible if people knew about the Centre in the first place. The interviews with Centre users illustrated that whilst people were aware of the service they were referred to, they often did not know what else the Centre provided. Given that the Centre aims to involve local people it was felt that there was a need to raise its profile in the area by providing leaflets, posters and other forms of information. The CAG suggested that they could collate information on the Centre and make it more readily available to local people and local voluntary and community groups. This was pursued, but no resources were provided to help with the production and distribution of the information.

Community involvement in the decision making process: In the interviews people pointed to the existence of the CAG as proof that community participation was active in the Centre. However, there were a number of criticisms made of the CAG. Some people felt that the way the CAG had been set up did not adequately reflect the Centre's aim of community participation. The existence on the 15 member CAG of three Centre staff members and all four professional members of the CMT led some people to believe that CAG could do no more than provide a forum for the discussion of issues between the seven lay representatives and the seven Centre staff and management representatives.

It was pointed out that when sensitive or controversial issues were raised, Centre staff members and management team members would attempt to explain and rationalize their position and defend their actions. This coupled with the staff and management's professional knowledge and experience often led to the lay members complying with the staff and management view. In the individual and group interviews, CAG members felt that this compliance reflected the imbalance of power that exists between those responsible for providing health care services and those that use them. Ultimately, people felt that this situation on CAG did not facilitate an equal partnership in the decision making process in the Centre.

Some of the community representatives interviewed felt that after three years of operation, CAG was still desperately trying to identify its role. It was not sure whether it was a 'decision maker', an 'advisory body' or a 'watchdog' and that its formal structure served to render it little more as a complaints forum with few direct powers to change or influence professional and/or managerial decisions.

The community representatives in CAG were criticized by some local community group representatives, Centre staff, GPs and managers for not being truly representative of the local community and for ultimately not being truly accountable to the local community for their actions. Whilst CAG members saw themselves as acting on behalf of the community they had no official mandate or obligation to report back to the local community. This raised for CAG the problem of identifying their role. Would they become decision makers and risk having their views compromised in the decision making process? Or, would they become a watchdog, and so avoid becoming an actual part of the decision making process but play an advisory role by commenting on and evaluating the decisions made by Centre staff, GPs and managers?

After the group interviews, a new CAG was elected and started work on redefining its role and devising a three year plan. The new CAG members also attempted to change the membership of the CAG to one which only has community and 'lay' representatives, with staff and Centre management invited to attend meetings to answer specific questions and points of clarification. The new CAT received a formal induction to the Centre and its work. These moves were regarded by some of the earlier critics of the CAG as a step in the right direction.

There was general agreement about the need to facilitate community involvement in the Centre. The post of community linkworker was felt to be one means of meeting this need. One person argued against having a 'community worker' as this could allow other workers involved in the Centre to abdicate their responsibility to encourage and facilitate more active community involvement. This issue arose in the group interviews and community representatives felt that a community linkworker or development worker would be only one part of the solution. Importantly though, they felt that if such a post was funded this would signal a commitment by resource managers a commitment to the aims of community participation.

In the group interviews with Centre staff and contracted GPs, it became clear that their understanding of community participation was somewhat limited. In general, Centre staff and GPs defined community participation as meaning working more closely with other PHC workers who were based in the community. They did not consider that it might mean the involvement of 'lay' people in the decision making process.

Some health authority managers interviewed felt that community involvement in the decision making process was inappropriate. They felt that whilst the health authority was interested in and concerned with promoting the concept of 'consumer sensitive' services, they were not ready to accept 'handing over the power to community management'. A local authority community worker expressed reservations about the ability of Centre staff and management to understand or implement community participation. Centre staff were mainly recruited from hospital settings and had little or no experience of working in community based settings in an equal partnership with local people. Management, too often made decisions based on their belief in their right to manage, rather than making decisions based on consultation and negotiation.

Conclusion

From the results of the evaluative study of the Lambeth Community Care Centre and the detailed assessment made of community particiation, a number of more general conclusions can be drawn. Whilst the aim of community participation is desirable, it faces a number of key definition problems. What is a community? What constitutes participation? Locally the impact of the Lambeth Community Care Centre's attempts at

216

community participation was restricted to the Centre itself. Little impact was made on the wider heath district, where community participation receives an even lower priority.

Politically, community participation was seen by resource managers (those responsible for managing finances) as being a low priority. For service managers (those responsible for the direct provision of services) it was a desirable concept, but one that was time consuming and difficult to put into practice without extra resources, staff and training to enable health workers to be more able to respond to the ideals of community participation.

Community participation also raised a dilemma for community representatives. Do they become compromised if they become part of the decision making process? Can they avoid this by formulating comments on and evaluating the decisions made? This dilemma has not yet been resolved in the case of Lambeth. However, it does point to an awkwardness in community participation that needs to be addressed.

Health care providers need to be trained in such a way as to enable them to provide a service more in partnership with those using or likely to use the services. This can be helped by exposing more health care workers who work in the secondary health care sector to local community and PHC settings.

The model of Lambeth Community Care Centre points to a possible blueprint for providing the right environment and services by which secondary health care workers can work in more local community based health care settings. This exposure can then help to redress the imbalances that arise between those who traditionally provide health services and those who use them.

Yugoslavia

Primary health care in Croatia

Since the beginning of the century, when the first concept of comprehensive PHC was introduced in Yugoslavia by the Andrija Stampar School of Public Health, there have been many phases in the development of the health system. The key units of the first health centre, founded in 1923, were departments for maternal and child care and preschool children, specific infectious diseases, a clinic for school medicine and a department for rural sanitation. The centre was mainly staffed by nurses and usually headed by a physician trained in preventive medicine. Staff were paid by the government, having salaries higher than average in private practice. The majority of GPs worked in private practice.

After World War II a central planning system was introduced. All health institutions were under the control of the central government with the majority of health care staff employed in the public sector. During the 1970s, a system of decentralisation and self management was introduced in health care, as well as in industry. In the late 1980s, the whole health system and PHC in particular began to change along with other political and social changes (multi-party parliament, privatisation, market economy). The early moves to a decentralised health care and insurance system and self management system is being centralised to a certain degree.

In Croatia some additional changes were introduced in 1991. Privatization of the health services was encouraged and supported by the government. Private services can be covered by basic health insurance. A personal/family GP based model of comprehensive PHC was promoted, although such a system was already traditional in certain parts of Croatia. There is free choice of PHC doctor. Pre-paid type of payment was introduced. The Ministry of Health is responsible for strategy, manpower planning and implementation, and is not obliged to accept all requests from local health authorities and health institutions as previously was the case. The parliament is now responsible for health policy, legislation and taxation. Whereas before, decisions on taxes for health care were made by the local 'self managing community of interest'.

PHC is organised around two types of institutions, the health centre ('Home of health') and the medical centre. The health centre provides ambulatory services and covers usually one commune (about 50,000 inhabitants). The health centre can also organize specialised clinics, usually for the prevalent health problems. Some outlying health centres have small maternity departments. The medical centre provides outpatient and inpatient services. The inpatient service is a general hospital with at least four departments (medicine, surgery, paediatric and gynaecology/obstetrics). The catchment area is between 70,000 to 150,000 inhabitants and functions as a health district. In large cities, teaching hospitals and health centres operate separately.

In Croatia, in 1988 there were 26 medical centres, 86 health centres, five teaching hospitals, 19 specialised hospitals and six public health institutes. The total number of beds were 7.5 per 1000 inhabitants; 4,001 physicians and 15,762 nursing staff worked in hospitals. Presently most of the physicians work in the public sector. In 1988 there was approximately one doctor for every 500 inhabitants. There are about 200 private physicians and dentists. General preventive measures and environmental control were organised by public health institutes on the four levels: federal, republic, regional and communal. Sanitary inspection was a part of overall government services and as such outside the health services.

In terms of general and health care system development, Yugoslavia once met the World Bank criteria as one of the 32 industrialised countries of the world. According to European criteria, it belonged to the group of developing countries, and on the basis of IPF criteria it was supported by UNDP funds. At the same time, Yugoslavia was seen by other developing countries as a model country which demonstrated a particular way of development. Now, of course, the situation is very different. However, the fragmentation of Yugoslavia and the turmoil created should not detract from its achievements in the field of health care.

Optimal development and utilisation of primary health care

Luka Kovacic and Ivan Stipanov

This project set out to assess the quality of PHC in the district of Zadar by analysing the efficiency, efficacy and accessibility of the care delivered. Three areas for investigation were identified: improve the access to an utilization of existing services; assess the communication linkages between types and levels of PHC; and examine the interface between primary and secondary care. The research encountered particular problems such that only a start on the first objective was made. Data collected to date gives a picture of the usage of the PHC services but it is not possible to come to any concrete observations and/or conclusions from the material.

Background

The district of Zadar consists of four communes: the town of Zadar and the three neighbouring areas of Benkovac, Biograd and Obrovac. The district contains rather heterogenous natural and geographic units: islands; coastal region and the Kotari; the hills of Benkovac; and, southern slopes of Velebit. The islands comprise about 16% of the entire area surface and nine percent of the population inhabits them.

According to the 1981 census there were 177,950 inhabitants in the district of Zadar. In the commune of Zadar the average yearly rate of population growth (1974-1981) was 0.8% and in the commune of Biograd 0.5%. Whereas in the commune of Benkovac and Obrovac the population declined by an average yearly rate of 0.6% and 0.8% respectively. At the same time, the number of households in all four communes increased. This was due to the breaking up of extended families and households with several generations as one of the consequences of the process of migration/urbanisation. The population of the district is ageing. In 1971 eight percent of the population was aged 65 and over and by 1981 this had risen to 10.2%.

The whole post World War II period has been characterised by a constant urbanisation process: migration of the inhabitants towards the commune centres, and especially to Zadar, whose population increased from 107,746 to 226,174 over the census period (1974-1981). With urbanisation has come a decline in the rural population. The agricultural households of the district had 80,674 inhabitants in 1961 (52.5% of the entire population). By 1981, this was down to 18 908, or only 11.6% of

220

the entire population.

Mortality and morbidity in the Zadar district was similar to that pertaining in Croatia as a whole. The one major difference was the low prevalence of carcinomas in the area, compared to Croatia. The five leading diseases or illnesses in the district of Zadar were: respiratory diseases (29.0%), nervous system & sensory organs diseases (11.3%), digestive system diseases (7.7%), skin diseases (7.5%), and muscular-skeletal diseases (7.1%).

PHC (provided by a network of over 30 units) organisationally was part of the medical centre based in Zadar. PHC was divided into general practice, occupational health, school medicine, dental health care and emergency service. The medical centre also included a general hospital and the psychiatric hospital in Zemunika. The psychiatric hospital on the island of Ugljan and the orthopaedic hospital in Biograd were independent institutions. The Republic Institute of Public Health in Zadar was engaged in environmental health, social medicine and epidemiology with microbiology. Health centres in Benkovac, Biograd and Obrovac provided PHC and some secondary health care through polyclinic-type work. Two outpatient departments were completely independent. These are the factory based occupational health outpatient departments.

The health needs of the whole district were provided from within the care of the medical centre and related specialized hospitals. For tertiary care the district population looked to the larger health centres in Zagreb, Split and Rijeka. Given the nature of the PHC system operating in the district of Zadar, it was decided to focus on the quality of the care delivered by analyzing the efficiency, efficacy and accessibility of health care. Initial discussions identified three areas for investigation:

*   appraisal and improvement of the accessibility and utilization of existing services;

*   assessment of the communication system between levels and types of primary health care;

*   examination of the interface between primary and secondary health care

Methodology

With regard to the first task, accessibility of PHC, the main issues seemed to be the need for a more prompt contact of patients with the first line of health care. In order to study the problem the following segments of PHC were chosen: general practice, school medicine, occupational health, general dental care and emergency health care. The elements considered were: geographical distance of the health care units from the patients; time distance with regard to public transportation; working hours of the PHC teams; choice of medical team; accessibility of telephone communication throughout 24 hours; and, organisation of emergency health care.

In the second task, (to analyse communication between segments of PHC), three issues were addressed:

* communication between occupational health and general practice;
* communication between occupational health and school medicine;
* communication between occupational health and dental health care.

It was considered of great significance to improve communication lines in order to increase the quality of health care, to reduce absenteeism and to rationalise the division of labour inside PHC.

The third task was related to the communication lines between primary and secondary health care. From everyday experience it was noted that in the Zadar district there was an increasing need for faster communication between primary and polyclinic-type secondary care. The results of polyclinic examinations rarely reached the PHC physicians on time and on occasions they did not reach them at all.

This communication problem was examined in two specialised outpatient departments: internal heart diseases and general surgery. The elements which were selected for investigation were: the organisation of polyclinic care; the waiting time for specialist's examination; the division of work between primary and secondary heath care; the expertise of teams in PHC; the motivation and stimulation for quality of work of PHC workers.

It was expected that by analysing this communication problem the cause of the deficiencies in communication lines between primary and secondary health care would be identified and resolved. Several evaluative methods were used in the study. These include participant observations, questionnaires and opinion surveys. During the implementation of the study, certain difficulties arose which resulted in delays to the project, such that it was only partially completed.

The two studies completed were an analysis of the utilisation of health care services in Zadar district, and a review of the accessibility of health care. Utilisation of health care services in Zadar district has increased

(Table 20) with all four communes reporting greater usage. However, looking at numbers or cases treated (Table 21), this reveals a mixed situation with increased usage in Benkovac and Obrovac and a decline in Biograd and Zadar. Why this should be so was difficult to discern but may be due in part to developments in health services not keeping pace with population growth in these two communes.

In terms of accessibility, given the structure of PHC in the district, it is not surprising to find that the direction of patient flow was from the other three communes into Zadar (Table 22).

Conclusion

This project offered great potential for evaluating the quality of PHC delivered by a centralised health care system. However, events conspired against the project to make it impossible to complete as originally conceived. The work done so far gives an indication of how and the way in which PHC facilities are being utilised in the district of Zadar. Given the current political climate prevailing in Croatia it is doubtful if the project ever will be concluded.

Table 20

The trends in the use of health care services

Region	Year (visits)	PHC (visits)	Polyclinics (visits)	Dental aids issued	Orthopaedic
Benkovac	1981	60,085	27,768	16,851	414
	1986	92,602	45,890	26,556	1,451
Biograd	1981	43,238	45,992	13,641	668
	1986	107,974	69,232	27,408	1,058
Obrovac	1981	117,637	26,483	7,423	230
	1986	178,463	54,200	27,941	887
Zadar	1981	781,818	755,003	150,302	4,242
	1986	905,138	1,066,370	234,2266	6,697

Source: Annual report of the Association of self-managing communities of interest in the field of health and health insurance of Croatia, different years.

Table 21
Number treated per 1000 users (public sector)

Region	Index 86/81	Average annual rate
Benkovac	134	6.03
Biograd	89	-2.30
Obrovac	292	23.90
Zadar	87	-2.75

Source: *Annual report of the Association of self-managing communities of interest in the field of health and health insurance of Croatia, different years.*

Table 22
Patients treated by type in Zadar medical centre

	Benkovac	*Biograd*	*Obrovac*	*Zadar*
All inpatients	963 (11%)	777 (9%)	504 (6%)	6563 (74%)
Specialist Outpatients	2674 (2%)	2829 (2%)	1715 (2%)	132123 (95%)
Diagnostic Procedures	5802 (4%)	3769 (2%)	2098 (1%)	150711 (93%)

Bibliography

Arnold, P., and Cole, I. (1987), 'The Decentralisation of Local Services: Rhetoric and Reality', in P. Hambleton and R. Hoggett (eds), *Decentrialization and democracy - Localising Public Services,* SAUS, Bristol.

Arnstein, S. (1969), 'A Ladder of Citizen Participation', *Journal American Institute of Planners*, 35 (7), pp. 216-244

Baric, L. (1990), 'A New Approach to Community Participation', *Journal of the Institute of Health Education*, 28 (2) pp. 41-42.

Betts, G., (1985), *Glyndon Ward Health Survey*, Greenwich Community Health Council, London.

Bichmann, W., Rifkin, S.B., Shrestha, M. (1989), 'Towards The Measurement of Community Participation,' *World Health Forum*, 10, pp. 467-476.

Birch, S., and Maynard, A. (1986), *The RAWP review: rawping primary care in the United Kingdom*, Paper 19, University of York, York.

Boaden, M., Goldsmith, M., Hampton, W., and Stringer, P. (1982), *Public Participation in Local Services*, Longman, Harlow.

Bone, H., Tromans, J.R., Taylor, J., (1988), *Healthy Heart and Lung Project*, Dudley Health Authority.

Buxton, M.J. and Klein, R.E. (1978), *Allocating health resources: commentary on the Report of the Resource Allocation Working Party*, Her Majesty's Stationary Office, London.

Calnan, M., Voulton, M., and Williams, T. (1986), *Health Education and GPs; A critical appraisal*, Health Services Research Unit, University of Kent, Canterbury.

Carnall, C.A. (1990), *Managing Change in Organisations*, Prentice Hall, Hemel Hempstead.

Cheema, G. and Rondinelli, D. (Eds), (1983), *Decentralization and Development*, Sage, London.

Corcoran, R., O'Shea, E. (1989), 'The placement of elderly persons: a logit estimation and cost analysis'. *The Economic and Social Review*, 20, pp. 219-41.

Culyer, A.J. (1980), *The political economy of social policy*, Martin Robertson, Oxford.

Curtis, S., (1983), *Intra-urban Variations in Health and Health Care. The Comparative Need for Health Care Survey of Tower Hamlets and Redbridge*. Vol.1. Adult Morbidity and Service Use. England: Health Research Group, Department of Geography and Earth Science, Queen Mary College.

Daley, G. (1987), 'Decentralisation: A new way of organising community health services', *Hospital and Health Services Review*. 83, pp. 72-74.

Dearden, R.W. (1985), '*Resources and health deprivation*', (Discussion paper 19), University of Birmingham, Birmingham.

Department of Health and Social Security, (1988), *Report of the NHS. Management Board Review of RAWP*. Department of Health and Social Security, London.

Dun, R., (1984), *The Relationship Between Occupational Class and Material Deprivation. The Experience of Physical Disability*, unpublished MSc dissertation. University of Southampton.

Dun, R., (1987), *Going Local? A study of West Lambeth District Health Authority*, Community Services Unit, West Lambeth Health Authority, London.

Dun, R., (1989), *Pictures of Health?*, A report of a community health survey carried out in Clapham, South London, Community Services Unit, West Lamberth Health Authority, London.

Dun, R., (1991), 'Working with the voluntary sector', in A. McNaught, (ed), *Managing Community Health Services*, Chapman and Hall, London.

Elcock, H. (1988), 'Alternatives to representative government in Britain: going local', *Public Policy and Administration* 3 (2) pp. 38-50.

Evans, E.O. and McBride, K. (1968) 'Hospital usage by a group practice', *Journal Royal College of General Practitioners*, 16, pp.294-306.

Fagence, M. (1977), *Citizen Participation in Planning*, Pergamon, Oxford.

Farquar, M., and Bowling, A. (1990), 'Preventative Activity', *Nursing Standard*, 4 (33), pp.54-55.

Farrant, W., and Taft, A. (1988), 'Building Healthy Public Policy in and Unhealthy Political Climate; A Case Study From North West Kensington' *Health Promotion International*, 3, pp.287-297.

Fullard E., Fowler G, and Gray M. (1987). 'Facilitating Prevention in Primary Health Care' in Heller, Bailey, Gott and Haures (eds), *Coronary Heart Disease: Reducing the Risk*, Open University Press, Milton Keynes.

Giraldes, M.R. (1987), *Equitative expenditure allocation in PHC services*, Thesis, National School of Public Health, Lisbon.

Giraldes, M.R. (1988), 'Equity and health expenditure', *Journal of Economic Studies*, VIII(4), July/September.

Giraldes, M.R. (1988), 'The equity principle in the allocation of health care expenditure on PHC services in Portugal: the human capital approach', *International Journal of Health Planning and Management*, 3, pp.167-183.

Giraldes, M.R. (1988), 'The allocation of resources in a public health system', *Analyse Social*, XXIV (101-102), pp. 815-828;

Giraldes, M.R. (1990), 'The equity and efficiency principle in the financing system of the NHS in Portugal', *Health Policy*, 14, pp. 13-28.

Godinho, J. (1990), 'Tipping The Balance Towards Primary Health Care; Managing Change At The Local Level', *International Journal of Health Planning And Management*, 15, pp.41-52.

Gott, M. (1986), *Training for Health Education and Promotion; The role of Doctors and Nurses*, Paper given at Education For Primary Health Care Conference, Oxford University.

Gott, M., and Warren, G. (1990), 'Neighbourhood health forums: local democracy at work, *World Health Forum*, 12, pp. 413-418.

Gray, D.P. (1979) 'The key to personal care', *Journal Royal College of General Practitioners*, 29, pp.666-678.

Green, A. (1987), 'Is There Primary Health Care in the UK?' *Health Policy and Planning*, 2 (2), pp. 129-137.

Grossman, M. (1972), *The demand for health: A theoretical and empirical investigation*, (Occasional Paper:119), National Bureau of Economic Research, XVII, New York.

Hambleton, P., and Hoggett, R. (eds) (1987), *Decentralisation and Democracy - Localising Public Services*, Occasional Paper 28, School of Advanced Urban Studies (SAUS), Bristol.

Hayes, M.V., and Manson Willms, S. (1990), 'Healthy Community Indicators: The perils of the search and the paucity of the find', *Health Promotion International*, 5(2), pp. 161-166.

Helenius, M., Marjamaki, P., Pekurinen, M. and Vohlonen, I. (1987) *Personal Doctor Program, Background, Objectives and Methods of the Finnish study*. Health Services Research by the National Board of Health in Finland 42. Valtion painatuskeskus, Helsinki.

Heller, Bailey, Gott and Haures (eds), (1987), *Coronary heart disease: reducing the risk*, Open University Press, Milton Keynes.

Henderson, G and Tarpey, M. (1990), *'Assessing the Lambeth Community Care Centre'* West Lambeth Health Authority, London.

HMSO (1984), *National Third Report of the Social Services Committee on Perinatal and Neonatal Mortality*, London: Her Majesty's Stationery Office.

Hunt, S., McKenna, S., McEwan, J., Papp, E., (1981), The Nottingham Health Profile. Subjective Health Status and Medical Consultations. *Social Science and Medicine*, 15A.

Jarman, B., (1983), 'Identification of underprivileged areas', *British Medical Journal*, 286, pp. 1705-9.

Johnson, Z., Dack, P., (1989), 'Small area mortality patterns', *Irish Medical Journal*, 82, pp 105-8.

Johnson, Z., Jennings, S., Fogarty, J., Johnson, H., Lyons, R., Doorly, P., Hynes, M., (1991), 'Behavioural risk factors among young adults in small areas with high mortality versus those in low mortality areas', *International Journal of Epidemiology*, 20, pp.989-96.

Kalimo, E., Hakkinen, U., Klaukka, T., Lehtonen, R. and Nyman, K. (1989) *Teitoja suomalaisten terveysturvasta*. Kansanelakelaitoksen julkaisuja M:67. Sosialiturvan tutkimuslaitos, Helsinki.

Kekki, P. (1982) Terveyskeskuksen laakaripalvelu - kaytto, sisalto ja hoidon jatkuvuus. *Suom Laadail* 37, pp. 2021-2027.

Kivell, P.T., Turton, B.J., and Dawson, B.R.P.(1990), 'Neighbourhoods For Health Service Administration', *Social Science and Medicine,* 30 (6), pp. 701-711.

Law, D. (1990), 'Sowing In The Care Patch', *Health Service Journal*, 99, p. 829.

Le Grand, J. (1982), *The strategy of equality. Redistribution and the social services*, George Allen & Unwin, London.

Le Grand, J. (1988). *Equity, health and health care*, VIII Journeys of Health Economics, May, Gran Canaria.

Levike (1989) *Suunnitelma vaestovastuuperiaatteen mukaisen toimintamallin kehittamisesta ja kayttoonotosta Leppavaaran palvelupiirissa*. Terveyskeskuslaakarin toyon kehittamisptojekti. Espoon terveysvirasto, Espoo.

Malcolm, L. (1989), 'Decentralisation Trends in the Management of New Zealand Health Services', *Health Policy*, 12(3) pp. 285-299.

Marklund, B., Bengtsson, C., (1989a), 'Medical advice by telephone at Swedish health centres. Who calls and what are the problems?' *Journal of Family Practice*, 6, pp 42-46.

Marklund, B., Silfveryhielm, B., Bengtsson, C., (1989b), 'Evaluation of an educational programme for telephone advisers in primary health care', *Family Practice*, 6, pp 263-7.

Marklund, B., Bengtsson, C., Bjorkander, E., (1990), 'Uniform guidance for medical care. A description of the process for preparing guidelines accepted by different levels of care', *Scandinavian Journal Caring Sciences*, pp 89-94.

Maynard, A. (1981), 'The inefficiency and inequalities of the health care systems of Western Europe', *Social Policy and Administration*, 15(2), pp.145-163.

Maynard, A. (1985), *The economics of addiction*, V Health Economics Conference, May, Lisbon.

Maynard, A. (1986), *Financing the UK National Health Service*, mimeo., University of York, York.

Maynard, A., and Ludbrook, A. (1983), *The allocation of health care resources in the United Kingdom*, mimeo., University of York, York.

McGuire, A., Henderson, J., and Mooney, G. (1988), *The economics of health care*, London: Routledge & Kegan Paul.

Mills, A., Vaughan, P., Smith, D., and Tabibzadeh, I. (1987), *Decentralization and Health For All Strategy*, World Health Organization, Geneva.

Mills, A., Vaughan, P., Smith, D., and Tabibzadeh, I. [eds], (1990), *Health System Decentralisation - Concepts, Issues and Country Experience*, WHO, Geneva.

Ministry of Health and Social Welfare (1986) - *Health for all by the year 2000. The Finnish national strategy*. Valtion painatuskeskus, Helsinki.

Mooney, G.H. (1983), 'Equity in health care: confronting the confusion', *effective Health Care*, 1, 179-184.

Nixon, L. (1986), *A Report from the Community Linkworker*. Lambeth Community Care Centre, West Lambeth Health Authority, London.

Olds, D.L. et al. (1986), 'Improving the delivery of prenatal care and outcomes of pregnancy: a randomised trial of nurse home visitation', *Paediatrics*, 77, pp. 16-28;

Organisation for Economic Cooperation and Development, (1990), *Health Care Systems in Transition - The Search for Efficiency*, Social Policy Studies, No.7, OECD, Paris.

Pateman, C. (1970) *Participation and Democratic Theory*, Cambridge University Press, Cambridge, p.71.

Paton, C. (1985), *The policy of resource allocation and its ramifications*, The Nuffield Provincial Hospitals Trust; London.

Pereira, J. (1988), *The economic interpretation of equity in health and health care*, VIII Journeys of Health Economics, Gran Canaria;

Peters, T. J., and Waterman, R. H. (1982), *In Search of Excellence - Lessons From America's Best Run Companies*, Harper & Row, New York.

Rathwell, T. (1987), *Strategic Planning in the Health Sector*, Croom Helm, London.

Rawls, K. (1972), *A theory of justice*, Oxford University Press; Oxford

Rifkin, S. B., Muller, F. and Bichmann, W. (1988), 'Primary Health Care; on measuring participation,' *Social Science and Medicine*: 9, pp. 931-940.

Scarpaci, J. (1991), 'Primary Care Decentralisation in the Southern Core: Shantytown Health Care as Urban Social Movement', *Annals of the Association of American Geographers*, 81(1) pp. 102-126.

Schieber, G., and Poullier, J.P. (1989), 'International Health Care Expenditure Trends: 1987', *Health Affairs* 1, pp. 169-177

Schwefel, D. (1985), *Economic instability, nutrition and health*, V Health Economics Conference, May, Lisbon.

Siler Wells, J. (1988), 'Strengthening Community Health Means Strengthening the Community', *Health Promotion* (Canada) 27, pp. 7-21.

Silvestre, A., Colomer, C., Nolasco, A., Gonzalez, L., and Alvarez-Dardet, C., (1990), 'Nivel de vida y estilos de vida: Hacia una ley de prevension inversa?' *Gacata Sanitaria*, 20, pp 189-92.

Simmie, J. (1974), *Citizens in Conflict : The Sociology of Town Planning*, Hutchinson, London.

Smith, G. and Cantley, C. (1985), *Assessing Health Care: a study in organisational evaluation*, Open University Press, MK, London.

Spratley, J. and Gott, M. (1988), *Education and Training For Health Promotion*. Report of a Feasibility Study. Dept of Health and Social Welfare, The Open University, Milton Keynes.

Steering Committee and Secretariat, (1989), *Fourth Workshop Report - Tipping The Balance Towards Primary Health Care*, November 18-22, Zadar, Yugoslavia.

Stillwell, B., Greenfield, S. Drury, M. and Hull, F. (1987), 'A nurse practitioner in general practice; working style and pattern of consultations', *Journal of the Royal College of Practitioners*, 37, pp. 154-7.

Townsend, P., Davidson, N., (eds), (1982), *Inequalities in Health*, The Black Report, Penguin, London.

Vohlonen, I. (1989) - *Personal doctor program, data, results and conclusions of the Finnish study.* Health Services Research by the National Board of Health in Finland, 50. Valtion painatuskeskus, Helsinki

Vuori, H. (1984), 'Primary Health Care in Europe; Problems and Solutions', *Community Medicine*, 6, pp. 221-231.

Whitehead, M., (1988), *The Health Divide. Inequalities in Health in the 1980s*, London, Penguin Books.

Williams, G.L. (1984), 'Observing and Recording Meetings', in Bell J. et al, *Conducting Small Scale Investigations in Educational Management.* Harper and Row, New York.

WMRHA (1983), *The West Midlands Regional Health Authority Report on Perinatal and Infant Mortality*, West Midlands Regional Health Authority, Birmingham.

World Health Organisation/United Nations Children's Fund, (1978), *Primary Health Care*, Report of the International Conference on Primary Health Care, Alma Ata, USSR, World Health Organisation, Geneva.

World Health Organization, (1980), *Formulating Strategies for Health For All By The Year 2000*, World Health Organization, Geneva.

World Health Organisation, (1985), *Targets for Health For All*, World Health Organisation, Regional Office for Europe, Copenhagen.

World Health Organisation, (1986), *Evaluation of the Strategy for Health for all by the year 2000*, Seventh Report on the world health situation, World Health Organisation, European Region, Copenhagen.

World Health Organisation, (1988a), *Priority Research for Health For All*, World Health Organisation, Regional Office for Europe, Copenhagen.

World Health Organisation, (1988b), *Research Policies for Health For All*, World Health Organisation, Regional Office for Europe, Copenhagen.

World Health Organisation, (1988c), *The Challenge of Implementation*, World Health Organisation, Geneva.

World Health Organisation, (1990), *Systems of Continuing Education: priority to district health personnel*, Technical Report Series. No 803, World Health Organisation, Geneva.

Wynn Williams, C. (1988), 'Coming to Grips with Groups', in Drennan V., *Health Visitors and Groups*. Heinemann Nursing, London.